GnRH ANALOGUES

The State of the Art 1993

GnRH ANALOGUES

The State of the Art
1993

*A Summary of the 3rd International Symposium
on GnRH Analogues in Cancer and
Human Reproduction, Geneva, February 1993*

EDITED BY BRUNO LUNENFELD
AND VACLAV INSLER

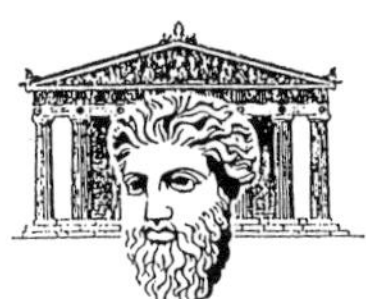

The Parthenon Publishing Group
International Publishers in Medicine, Science & Technology

Casterton Hall, Carnforth,
Lancs LA6 2LA, UK

One Blue Hill Plaza, Pearl River,
New York 10965, USA

Published in the UK and Europe by
The Parthenon Publishing Group Ltd.
Casterton Hall
Carnforth, Lancs. LA6 2LA

Published in North America by
The Parthenon Publishing Group Inc.
One Blue Hill Plaza
PO Box 1564, Pearl River
New York 10965, USA

Typeset by AMA Graphics Ltd., Preston, Lancashire
Printed and bound in Great Britain by
Redwood Books, Trowbridge, Wiltshire

Contents

Editorial Note

Throughout the text the numbers shown in brackets – for example [39] – refer to the original abstract numbers as published in *Gynecological Endocinology*, **7**, Supplement 2, 1993 (which was the Book of Abstracts for *The 3rd International Symposium on GnRH Ananlogues in Cancer and Human Reproduction*).

At the end of each chapter, after the references, a bibliography is provided which lists in full the abstracts quoted in that chapter. This bibliography follows the order in which the abstracts are referred to in the chapter and the numbers do not, therefore, necessarily appear in numerical sequence.

List of principal contributors

G. Benagiano
University of Rome 'La Sapienza'
First Institute of Obstetrics and
    Gynecology
Policlinico Umberto 1
00161 Rome
Italy

M. Breckwoldt
Universitäts Frauenklinik
Hugstetter Straße 55
7800 Freiburg
Germany

K. Bühler
Center for Reproductive Medicine
Kaiserstraße 5–7
66111 Saarbrücken
Germany

V. Insler
Department of Obstetrics and
    Gynecology
Kaplan Hospital
Rehovot
Israel

R. Kauli
Institute of Pediatric and Adolescent
    Endocrinology
Beilinson Medical Center
Petah Tikva 49100
Israel

L. Kiesel
Universitäts Frauenklinik
Schleichstraße 4
D-7400 Tübingen
Germany

F. Labrie
CHUL Research Center and Laval
    University
2705 Laurier Boulevard
Québec G1V 4G2
Canada

B. Lunenfeld
Department of Life Sciences
Bar-Ilan University
Ramat-Gan
Israel

K. S. Moghissi
Department of Obstetrics and
    Gynecology
Wayne State University School of
    Medicine
Hutzel Hospital
4707 St. Antoine Boulevard
Detroit
Michigan 48201
USA

Z. Naor
Department of Biochemistry
The George S. Wise Faculty of Life
    Sciences
Tel Aviv University
Ramat Aviv 69978
Israel

J. Rivier
The Clayton Foundation Laboratories
    for Peptide Biology
The Salk Institute
La Jolla
California 92037
USA

Preface

To take stock of the state of the art in this fast-moving field, International Symposia on GnRH Analogues in Cancer and Human Reproduction were held in Geneva in 1988, 1990 and 1993. These symposia permitted frank interdisciplinary discussions and the exchange of results as well as the development of ideas. The interdisciplinary nature of this field of research became evident from the 140 lectures presented on basic and clinical features of GnRH analogues during the 1993 symposium.

These lectures were grouped into nine sections, each of which was covered by an established international authority in his/her specific field and summarized in the form of state-of-the-art lectures.

For the benefit of the participants and for those who could not join us, these state-of-the-art lectures are reproduced in the form of this book. It is our hope that the chosen raporteurs have presented in this volume the state of the art of GnRH analogues '1993'. The book, although small in size, summarizes clearly the manifold impact of GnRH analogues in the management of many pathological conditions and may open new dimensions for students, physicians, biochemists and researchers. We also hope it will stimulate you and your colleagues to join us at the 4th Symposium, 8–11 February, 1996.

The rapid publication of this volume would not have been possible without the continuous help of the contributors, the encouragement of the International Scientific Committee, the Secretariat, Parthenon Publishing and the generous contributions of many sponsors.

May 1993   *Bruno Lunenfeld, MD, FRCOG, FACOG (Hon.)*
Vazlav Insler, MD, FRCOG

Prologue

M. Breckwoldt

This book reflects the rapid development in the field of GnRH, GnRH agonists and antagonists in basic science and their clinical applications. All aspects associated with the use of GnRH analogues are covered in the form of comprehensive state-of-the-art papers based on a large quantity of recent data presented at the Third International Symposium on GnRH Analogues in Cancer and Human Reproduction, Geneva, Switzerland, 1993. Therefore, the volume provides detailed and up-to-date information in a concentrated form. The following topics are presented:

(1) Novel antagonists – physicochemical properties, pharmacological activities, efficacy in the human.

(2) Mechanism of action of GnRH upon gonadotropin release and synthesis.

(3) GnRH agonists in the treatment of female infertility.

(4) GnRH agonists in the management of endometriosis.

(5) GnRH analogues in the management of leiomyomas.

(6) GnRH agonists in precocious puberty and small-growing children.

(7) GnRH agonists in prostate cancer.

(8) GnRH agonists in the treatment of cancer of the breast and the reproductive organs.

(9) GnRH agonists and safety.

Considering the fact that the 'castration effect' of GnRH agonists was discovered in 1978, it is amazing to note that their clinical usefulness and many forms of application have almost become routine in such a short period.

1

Novel antagonists of GnRH: a compendium of their physicochemical properties, activities, relative potencies and efficacy in humans

J. Rivier

INTRODUCTION

I have been given by Professor B. Lunenfeld, whom I gratefully acknowledge, the opportunity to summarize one of the most exciting aspects of gonadotropin releasing hormone (GnRH) pharmacology. In two words, I am to extract, from a series of presentations entitled 'GnRH antagonists', the salient characteristics of newly disclosed GnRH antagonists that are likely to become 'the drugs of the future' when it comes to the management of sexual steroid-dependent pathophysiologies, induction of ovulation and contraception.

In order to be used for any of the above-mentioned conditions and certainly much more so as fertility regulators in humans, GnRH antagonists must be extremely potent, long-acting, and exhibit negligible side-effects such as the stimulation of histamine release. In order to be commercially viable, these analogues also need to meet rigorous criteria, such as being easy to formulate for acute or slow release and economical to make.

Table 1 shows the structures and potencies (antiovulatory and histamine release) of all analogues disclosed at this meeting which are presently in clinical use or with the potential of being available for clinical use. They are presented in the order of their increased ability to release histamine. As can be seen, antiovulatory data in an aqueous buffer are presented; they reflect the ability of these analogues to inhibit gonadal functions.

Table 1 Structure, trade name, antiovulatory and histamine-releasing activities of GnRH analogues

Compounds	Name	Activities*
[Ac-DCpa^{1,2},DBta^3,DLys^6,DAla^{10}]GnRH	ORG 30850 [21]	NA
[Ac-DNal^1,DCpa^2,DPal^3,Arg^5,DGlu^6(AA),DAla^{10}]GnRH	Nal-Glu [6, 10, 17, 21]	0.5 (8/16)
		His: 2.0
[Ac-DNal^1,DCpa^2,DPal^3,DCit^6,DAla^{10}]GnRH	SB-75 [6, 11, 12, 15, 17, 20, 22]	2.0 (0/8)
	Cetrorelix	His: 2.1
[Ac-DNal^1,DCpa^2,DPal^3,DHar^6(Ng,Ng^{1}Et$_2$),Har^8,(Ng,Ng^{1}Et$_2$),DAla^{10}]GnRH	RS-26306 [6, 9]	2.5 (0/8)
	Ganirelix	His: 11
[Ac-DNal^1,DCpa^2,DPal^3,N$^\alpha$MeTyr^5,DLys^6(Nic),ILys^8,DAla^{10}]GnRH	A-75998 [6, 7]	4.0 (3/8)
		His: 22
[Ac-DNal^1,DCpa^2,DPal^3,N$^\alpha$CH$_3$Aph^5(atz),DAph^6(atz),ILys^8,DAla^{10}]-GnRH	Azaline C [6]	1.0 (2/8)
		His: 72
[Ac-DNal^1,DCpa^2,DPal^3,DHCit^6,ILys^8,DAla^{10}]GnRH	EP24332 [14, 17]	2.0 (CI)
	Antarelix	His: 81
[Ac-D3Qal^1,DCpa^2,DPal^3,Lys^5(cisPzACAla),DLys^6(Pic),ILys^8,DAla^{10}]-GnRH	Lystide [5]	1.0 (1/8)
		His: 171
[Ac-DNal^1,DCpa^2,DPal^3,Aph^5(atz),DAph^6(atz),ILys^8,DAla^{10}]-GnRH	Azaline B [6, 17]	1.0 (0/7)
		His: 224
[Ac-DNal^1,DCpa^2,DPal^3,Lys^5(Nic),DLys^6(Nic),ILys^8,DAla$^{10]}$-GnRH	Antide [5, 6, 8, 16]	8.0 (2/8)
		His: > 300

* Antiovulatory assay in about 1% DMSO: dosage in μg/rat (rats ovulating/total); His = histamine: ED_{50}, expressed in μg/ml, is an estimate of the molar concentration at which the peptides release 50% of the maximum releasable histamine from rat peritoneal mast cells. ED_{50} for GnRH is 186; NA, not available; CI, complete inhibition

Table 2 Biological and physical properties of GnRH antagonists

	*High potency**	*Long action*[†]	*High solubility*[‡]	*Low histamine***	*Gelling*[††]
Nal–Glu	yes	no	yes	no	no
Antide	yes	yes	no	yes	yes
SB-75	yes	yes	yes	no	no
RS-26306	yes	yes	yes	no	yes
Azaline B	yes	yes	yes	yes	yes
Azaline C	yes	no	yes	no	yes
A-75998	no	no	yes	no	no

*Complete inhibition of ovulation at 2.5 µg/rat or less in at least one vehicle; [†]greater than 48 h after 50 µg subcutaneous injection in castrated male rats; [‡]greater than 10 mg/ml at a pH of 5.0 or above with low viscosity; **ED_{50} higher than that of GnRH; [††]gels after subcutaneous injection in an aqueous vehicle at 10 mg/ml

Table 2 presents a qualitative evaluation of some of these analogues when it comes to their ability to inhibit ovulation, to release histamine , and to be soluble at the concentrations required for short-term and long-term administration. Some of these analogues will form gels after administration, a property that does not necessarily correlate with the fact that some of these peptides are extremely long acting *in vivo* when others exhibit rather transient activities[1]. It should be noted that the ideal analogue would be extremely potent and, if at all possible, would be ten times as potent as the presently available analogues; it would exhibit long duration of action and high solubility in aqueous buffers, it would be inactive in its ability to release histamine and would not gel under the conditions mentioned in the legend of Table 2.

ANALOGUE DESIGN

Potency in the antiovulatory assay

Potencies for the different analogues are presented in Table 1. All analogues have slightly different potencies. It may not be apparent from this table but one of the conclusions reached at this meeting was that the potency of an analogue is dependent on the solvent in which it has been injected. Hydrophilic peptides are significantly more effective in inhibiting ovulation in an aqueous buffer than are hydrophobic peptides. Conversely, hydrophobic peptides have the same ability to inhibit ovulation at about the same low dose whether administered in corn oil or polyethylene glycol.

Duration of action

Duration of action is another critical property of an analogue which was discussed. It is noteworthy that all antagonists tested[1] had different profiles when administered intravenously. It was noted that such a property may or may not be useful depending on the desired end effect and the nature of the delivery system. Any scenario is conceivable and probably achievable in view of the fact that none of the antagonists had identical half-lifes in the *in vivo* system where they were tested (Rivier *et al.*)[6]. No real consensus was really reached as to whether an 'ideal GnRH antagonist' should or should not be long-acting.

Solubility and ability to form gels

It is generally admitted that the solubility of a compound in a particular solvent (g/l) is a constant. In the case of peptides, this notion was challenged. Indeed, it may be surprising to know that a peptide can be very easily solubilized in an aqueous buffer. It may further remain in solution for an indefinite period of time. However, it is not at all unusual (and this is the case for most of the GnRH antagonists developed so far) that the peptide, which first assumed a random conformation in solution, has slowly rearranged to yield a significant and critical concentration of an ordered and less soluble conformer which suddenly gels. In the case of GnRH, it was suggested that the stabilized form consisted of beta sheets which are known to aggregate and be less soluble. It was suggested that those gels (not to be confused with the precipitated form of a peptide which would assume an unordered conformation) may be a useful form of the peptides when it comes to devising new delivery systems. The contribution by Haviv *et al.* [7] clearly demonstrated that the introduction of a methyl group on the backbone nitrogen of residue 5 would result in an analogue that is significantly more soluble in aqueous buffers. This observation was confirmed by Rivier *et al.* [6], who introduced that modification in Azaline C. It is unfortunate that such a favorable modification when it comes to solubility also results in the loss of some potency in the antiovulatory assay and in significantly greater ability of the peptides to release histamine.

Histamine-releasing activity

The histamine-releasing activity of the analogues clinically investigated was on the minds of many participants. It was noted that some peptides, such as the MCD peptide, have an ED_{50} of 2×10^{-8}, somatostatin has an ED_{50} of 1.5×10^{-6}, while GnRH with an ED_{50} of 1.3×10^{-4}, is considerably less potent. While many of the analogues presented in Table 1 (including the Nal–Glu antagonist, which has been extensively studied in clinical settings) have ED_{50}s smaller than that of GnRH, a few antagonists are considerably safer with ED_{50}s greater than that of GnRH. While most participants at the meeting agreed that this property of GnRH antagonists was not desirable, no consensus was reached as to what could be considered safe and what could not. The point, made by a few, that, since it is possible to obtain antagonists with very low histamine-releasing activity, all future drug candidates should belong to that category, was in general well taken despite the fact that it was also suggested that, for certain indications, the risk : benefit ratio is such that low levels of histamine-releasing activity may be acceptable. The point, that GnRH superagonists (considered to be safe) have an ED_{50} of around 40 µg/ml and that equivalent antagonists should, therefore, also be safe, did not take into consideration the fact that the antagonists will have to be administered at doses at least ten times greater than those at which the superagonists are given in order to be effective. A unique contribution by Gordon *et al.* [21] demonstrated that the *in vivo* histamine-releasing effects of GnRH antagonists result in prolactin secretion. It was shown that the release of prolactin by the antagonists was uniquely due to their ability to release histamine, since antihistamine inhibited this response in parallel studies.

Cyclic analogues

Data on cyclic analogues of GnRH with potencies equal to that of the most potent (as measured by antiovulatory assay) linear analogues were presented [6]. At this time, however, there is no evidence that these analogues have any of the properties that were expected from these constrained analogues. It was hypothesized that cyclic analogues would ultimately be resistant to degradation (which they are, but not necessarily to any greater extent than the linear analogues), and that they would be orally active. Here again, no evidence was presented that this was the case. Because these cyclic analogues have defined conformations[2,3], it was postulated that knowledge of the bioactive conformation of GnRH antagonists would help in the design of non-peptide ligands, which would have such desired properties as being orally active. It was suggested that this approach and its success may be the 'light at the end of the tunnel' when it comes to the development of peptido-mimetics interacting with the GnRH receptor.

CLINICAL INVESTIGATIONS

Biological actions of GnRH antagonists

When it comes to the use of GnRH antagonists in the clinic, Nal–Glu has had an early start[4–15]. While the basic principles governing gonadotropin secretion in men and women were elucidated using the Nal–Glu antagonist, it is encouraging to see that numerous other and safer analogues are being at present developed. In order to be nearly 100% effective, doses ranging from 5 to 10 mg per individual had to be administered. Formulations (content and concentration in active ingredient) were generally not disclosed and considered proprietary.

Inhibition of LH and FSH

GnRH antagonists inhibit luteinizing hormone (LH) and follicle stimulating hormone (FSH) secretion; of interest was the observation that, while the inhibition of LH is rapid in onset, that of FSH is not as immediate, although in long-term treatment it is also very profound[8–10]. What is also of some interest is that in humans full suppression of LH is not necessary to obtain very low levels of testosterone.

In vitro fertilization

Drs Bouchard [10] and Diedrich [11] presented results clearly indicating that the use of GnRH antagonists in combination with human menopausal gonadotropins for induction of ovulation may be important. While Dr Bouchard worked with Nal–Glu, Dr Diedrich used SB-75. From Table 1 it can be surmised that both analogues are very similar and, because of their relatively high potency at releasing histamine, may not be the best candidates for this particular application.

Anti-tumor activity

Dr Reissmann and colleagues [15] tested the anti-tumor activity of SB-75 in rats bearing estrogen-dependent DMBA-induced mammary tumors. Within the range of 31.6–360 µg/kg daily, a significant tumor regression was obtained. The anti-tumor effect and long-lasting tumor growth inhibition were also observed after subcutaneous injection of single high doses of SB-75 (1–10 mg/kg). In these experiments, the luteinizing hormone releasing hormone (LHRH) antagonist Antide was less effective in the induction of tumor regression and its duration of action was shorter. A permanent anti-tumor response was also achieved with a dose of 1 mg/kg given subcutaneously once a week. Even after a treatment period of 140 days, the suppression of tumor growth was maintained, indicating no induction of tolerance. I think that all these points (doses, mode of administration, duration of action and no induction of tolerance) are extremely important if any one antagonist of GnRH is ever going to be used to treat cancers. *In vitro*, Drs Karas [12], using SB-75, and Motta [13], using a GnRH superagonist and somatostatin, presented inhibitory effects of these peptides on cancer cell growth.

Contraception

Dr Nieschlag presented some very interesting results in monkeys. Tested in orchidectomized monkeys, SB-75, Azaline B and Antarelix were found to be more potent than Nal–Glu and Antide in their antigonadotropic effects [17].

Dr Sommer and colleagues [20] reported on the effect of administration of SB-75 in normal women and showed that this antagonist is indeed potent. This was in contradistinction with the work of Porchet and colleagues [8] who found very disappointing results after intravenous administration of Antide in healthy males. This same antagonist, Antide, reported to produce prolonged inhibition of gonadotropin secretion in ovariectomized monkeys by Nieschlag and colleagues [17], was also tested in the rat by Aubert and colleagues [16], who found it to be also quite effective. The poor and disappointing results obtained with Antide in humans remained a puzzling mystery.

Where and when ever reported, the effects of short-term as well as medium-term administration of the GnRH antagonists were reversible.

CONCLUSIONS

It can, therefore, be surmised that the success of a GnRH antagonist in clinical use may depend on the ability of its promoter/sponsor to develop the right formulation with the right analogue. Preliminary results suggest that the properties of the formulated antagonists should not be expected to be identical to that of the non-formulated materials. In that vein, a very important breakthrough was the report that Ganirelix has been formulated in a form that allows sustained concentrations of 20 ng/ml for 28 days in the human.

When the question came as to what was to be expected in the future, there was in general, great optimism. It was not clear for lack of enough clinical data, despite the fact that each group had great faith in the future of their antagonist, whether any of the compounds described at this conference will ever become drugs. It was my appreciation, however, that, because GnRH antagonists in contradistinction with the agonists, inhibit gonadotropin secretion immediately upon administration and because the degree of inhibition is more profound, such compounds will be extensively used in the years to come, not only in an academic setting but also with the aim of developing a drug. Last but not least, we as chemists are still faced with problems of formulation, and probably cost-effectiveness.

The future is bright: we expect to develop orally active molecules sometime in the future and, as far as I am concerned, they will probably be derived from knowledge of GnRH's bioactive conformation and the rational design of peptido-mimetics.

ACKNOWLEDGEMENTS

I thank Dr M. Karten from the Contraceptive Development Branch, Center for Population Research NICHD for obtaining most of the antiovulatory analyses and histamine release activities described in Table 1 as well as for the results from gelling studies reported in Table 2. Research was performed under NICHD contract NO1-HD-3-31-71

DISCUSSION

Prof. B. Lunenfeld   In which clinical situation would there be an advantage for the antagonist over the agonist?

Dr J. Rivier   I am certainly not the most qualified person to answer; however, I would think that an antagonist would be extremely beneficial in any circumstance where immediate and profound inhibition of gonadotropin is required.

Answer from the floor   If a safe antagonist were available, it would offer considerable advantage over the agonists we have at the present time. For example, let us address the question of the myoma of the uterus. We have patients who have large myoma, and who present with heavy bleeding. We want an immediate effect. We do not want the stimulatory phase (which may last as long as 3–4 weeks) of the agonist. An antagonist would definitely be an advantage in such a situation. Dysfunctional uterine bleeding is another situation. There are other fields in clinical medicine, IVF perhaps being one. So, I believe that there are definite indications in clinical medicine where the antagonist would offer a significant advantage.

Dr Haviv   I am wondering whether the ED_{50} in the histamine release assay is a good indication of how the compound will perform clinically? More specifically, we have seen that SB-75, which has an ED_{50} of around 2.0 µg/ml, has not had any major problem clinically. Can you comment?

Dr Rivier   I am concerned with one aspect of your question and that is that 'there was no major problem' observed with the use of SB-75. Here I want to emphasize the word *'major'*. At this time, while I do not think that any of the analogues described at this meeting (see Table 1) will be used as contraceptives, I still believe that the field cannot afford *any* problems, be they major, minor, or inexistent. You have now to balance this answer, based on principles, with reality, where, in life-threatening cases, a mild erythema may be accepted.

Dr Haviv   I agree with you because, as indicated also in this meeting, the formation of edema is not dose-dependent, in which case I wonder whether it is related to histamine.

Dr Rivier While this side-effect does not seem to be dose-dependent, it is unfortunately peptide-dependent. Some peptides will release prolactin and some others will not [21]. If prolactin release is a measure of the release of histamine, then those compounds that release prolactin should be questioned.

Prof. Lunenfeld Dr Rivier, if I understand you correctly, you imply that a regulatory agency will distinguish peptides on the basis of their ability to release histamine in such a way that a compound from Class X could be for contraception, a compound from Class Y could be used for life-threatening diseases and a compound from Class Z could be used for *in vitro* fertilization and other situations.

Dr Rivier I cannot talk for the Federal Food and Drug Administration (FDA) or any regulatory agency.

Prof. Lunenfeld No, I was just wondering whether that was what you were suggesting when you made the distinction between life-threatening situations and contraception.

Dr Rivier Before I answer that question, I will raise another question myself. 'In the long-term, what do you think the role or the effect of such amino acids as pyridylalanine, amino-triazolyl-phenylalanines, para-chloro-phenylanines and naphthylalanines will be?' One would expect that all those amino acids may accumulate over some time. While there is evidence that some of the peptides described here do not seem to degrade easily, it will turn out to be a concern of the regulatory agencies. I have not answered your question and I have made the story that much more complicated. However, I think that the US FDA has always been extremely reasonable and has taken the whole development of the analogues case by case, one after the other. They have looked at the protocols that were proposed and decided that they were safe, and have given the go-ahead. I think that we have had, in this area, a very positive attitude.

Prof. Lunenfeld   Do you see any possibility of having any antagonists without unnatural amino acids in the future – the near future?

Dr Rivier   The answer is 'Yes', if you delete all the amino acids and make it another drug, such as a peptido-mimetic derived from our studies with cyclic analogue. You will not have any unnatural amino acids any more, but you will have an unnatural drug!

REFERENCES

1. Rivier, J., Porter, J., Hoeger, C., Theobald, P., Craig, A. G., Dykert, J., Corrigan, A., Perring, M., Hook, W. A., Siraganian, R. P., Vale, W. and Rivier, C. (1992). Gonadotropin releasing hormone antagonists with Nω-triazolyl-ornithine, -lysine or -para-aminophenylalanine residues at positions 5 and 6. *J. Med. Chem.*, **35**, 4270–8
2. Rizo, J., Koerber, S. C., Bienstock, R. J., Rivier, J., Hagler, A. T. and Gierasch, L. M. (1992). Conformational analysis of a highly potent, constrained gonadotropin-releasing hormone antagonist. 1. Nuclear magnetic resonance. *J. Am. Chem. Soc.*, **114**, 2852–9
3. Rizo, J., Koerber, S. C., Bienstock, R. J., Rivier, J., Gierasch, L. M. and Hagler, A. T. (1992). Conformational analysis of a highly potent, constrained gonadotropin-releasing hormone antagonist. 2. Molecular dynamics simulations. *J. Am. Chem. Soc.*, **114**, 2860–71
4. Pavlou, S. N., Rivier, J., Vale, W. and Kamilaris, T. (1990). Clinical pharmacology of LHRH antagonists. In Vickery, B. H. and Lunenfeld, B. (eds.) *Precocious Puberty, Contraception and Safety Issues*, Vol. IV; pp. 127–31. (Dordrecht: Kluwer Academic Publishers)
5. Pavlou, S. N., Brewer, K., Farley, M. G., Lindner, J., Bastias, M. -C., Rogers, B. J., Rivier, J. E., Swift, L. L., Vale, W. W., Conn, P. M. and Herbert, C. M. (1991). Combined administration of a GnRH antagonist and testosterone in men induces reversible azoospermia without loss of libido. *J. Clin. Endocrinol. Metab.*, **73**, 1360–9
6. McGrath, G. A., Goncalvez, R., Udupa, J., Grossman, R. L., Pavlou, S. N., Molitch, M. E., Rivier, J., Vale, W. W. and Snyder, P. J. (1993). New technique for quantitation of pituitary adenoma size: use in evaluating treatment of gonadotroph adenomas with a GnRH antagonist. *J. Clin. Endocrinol., Metab.*, in press
7. Kolp, L. A., Pavlou, S. N., Urban, R. J., Rivier, J. E., Vale, W. W. and Veldhuis, J. D. (1992). Abrogation by a potent gonadotropin-releasing hormone antagonist of the estrogen progesterone-stimulated surge-like release of luteinizing hormone

and follicle-stimulating hormone in postmenopausal women. *J. Clin. Endocrinol. Metab.*, **75**, 993–7

8. Salameh, W., Bhasin, S., Steiner, B. S., McAdams, L. A., Peterson, M., Rivier, J. E., Vale, W. W. and Swerdloff, R. S. (1990). Marked suppression of gonadotropins and testosterone by an antagonist analog of gonadotropin-releasing hormone in men. *Fertil. Steril.*, **55**, 156–64

9. Tom, L., Bhasin, S., Salameh, W., Steiner, B., Peterson, M., Sokol, R. Z., Berman, N., Rivier, J., Vale, W. and Swerdloff, R. S. (1992). Induction of azoospermia in normal men with combined Nal–Glu gonadotropin-releasing hormone (GnRH) antagonist and testosterone enanthate. *J. Clin. Endocrinol. Metab.*, **75**, 476–83

10. Bagatell, C. J., McLachlan, R. I., de Kretser, D. M., Burger, H. G., Vale, W. W., Rivier, J. E. and Bremner, W. J. (1989). A comparison of the suppressive effects of testosterone and of a new, potent GnRH antagonist on gonadotropin and inhibin levels in normal men. *J. Clin. Endocrinol. Metab.*, **69**, 43–8

11. McLachlan, R. I., Cohen, N. L., Vale, W. W., Rivier, J. E., Burger, H. G., Bremner, W. J. and Soules, M. R. (1989). The importance of LH in the control of inhibin and progesterone secretion by the human corpus luteum. *J. Clin. Endocrinol. Metab.*, **68**, 1078–85

12. Tenover, J. S., Dahl, K. D., Vale, W. W., Rivier, J. E. and Bremner, W. J. (1990). Hormonal responses to a potent gonadotropin hormone-releasing antagonist in normal elderly men. *J. Clin. Endocrinol. Metab.*, **71**, 881–8

13. Bagatell, C. J., Knopp, R. H., Vale, W. W., Rivier, J. E. and Bremner, W. J. (1992). Physiologic testosterone levels in normal men suppresses high-density lipoprotein cholesterol levels. *Ann. Intern. Med.*, **116**, 967–73

14. Ditkoff, E. C., Cassidenti, D. L., Paulson, R. J., Sauer, M. V., Wellington, L. P., Rivier, J., Yen, S. S. C. and Lobo, R. A. (1992). The gonadotropin-releasing hormone antagonist (Nal–Glu) acutely blocks the luteinizing hormone surge but allows for resumption of folliculogenesis in normal women. *Am. J. Obstet. Gynecol.*, **165**, 1811–17

15. Roseff, S. J., Kettel, L. M., Rivier, J., Burger, H. G., Baulieu, E. and Yen. S. S. C. (1990). Accelerated dissolution of luteal-endometrial integrity by the administration of antagonists of GnRH and progesterone to late luteal phase women. *Fertil. Steril.*, **54**, 805–10

BIBLIOGRAPHY

Abstracts of relevant papers presented at the 3rd International Symposium on GnRH Analogues in Cancer and Human Reproduction.

5. Three stages of antagonists of LHRH. K. Folkers, C. Bowers, A. Janecka, T. Janecki, USA

6. Linear and cyclic analogs of GnRH. Are we seeing the light at the end of the tunnel? J. Rivier, L. Gierasch, J. Rizo, S. Koerber, A. Hagler, W. Vale, C. Rivier, USA

7. GnRH antagonists containing NMeTry[5]. F. Haviv, T. D. Fitzpatrick, C. J. Nichols, R. E. Swenson, N. A. Mort, E. N. Bush, G. Diaz, A. T. Nguyen, V. A. Cybulski, J. A. Leal, G. Bammert, N. S. Rhutasel, P. W. Dodge, E. S. Johnson, J. Knittle, J. Greer, USA

8. Clinical pharmacology of antide after intravenous administration in 8 healthy male volunteers. H. C. Porchet, V. Beltrami, J. -Y le Cotonnec, Switzerland

9. Rapid suppression of testicular and ovarian function by daily subcutaneous (SC) administration of ganirclix (GAN), a GnRH antagonist. S. E. Monroe, R. B. Jaffe, S. N. Pavlou, M. R. Henzi, USA

10. GnRH antagonist administration during the periovulatory period prevents LH surges in normal women: a possible role for GnRH antagonists in controlled ovarian stimulation. P. Bouchard, S. Dubourdieu, R. Frydman, B. Charbonnel, France

11. Induction of ovulation for *in vitro* fertilization controlled by GnRH-antagonist cetrorelix administered in combination with human menopausal gonadotrophins. K. Diedrich, D. Klingmuller, R. Reismann, Germany

12. Inhibition of endometrial and breast cancer cell growth by the GnRH antagonist, SB-75, is associated with increased release of IGF-binding proteins, M. Karas, M. Marbach, D. Kleinman, E. Hershkovitz, E. Bosin, D. LeRoith, J. Levy, Israel

13. Human prostatic carcinoma cells direct effect of LHRH agonists and of somatostatin. M. Motta, Italy

14. Further studies on antarelix (EP24332), a water soluble LHRH antagonist. R. Deghenghi, F. Boutignon, P. Wuthrich, V. Lenaerts, A. Caraty, P. Bouchard, France

15. Hormone suppressive and antitumor activity of cetrorelix a new LH-RH antagonist. T. Reissmann, P. Hilgard, J. Engel, A. M. Comaru-Schally, A. V. Schally, Germany, USA

16. Mechanism of action of the GnRH antagonist antide for the long term inhibition of gonadotropin secretion in the rat. M. L. Aubert, S. L. Li, B. Vuagnat, A. Eshkol, P. C. Sizonenko, Switzerland

17. GnRH antagonists (ANT) in men and non-human primates: towards the development of male contraception. E. Nieschlag, G. F. Weinbauer, H. M. Behre, Germany

18. Effect of GnRH antagonist (TX51) on ovarian plasminogen activator activity in rats. Y. Wang, J. -S, Qiu, J. -F Dai, W. Li, China *(Not presented)*

19. Effect of the GnRH-antagonist triptorelin on serum-lipoproteins in normolipemic male volunteers. K. A. Brensing, D. Klingmuller, C. H. Kinast, K. von Bergmann, Germany

20. Effect of the GnRH antagonist cetrorelix in normal women. L. Sommer, K. Diedrich, D. Klingmuller, Germany

21. Systemic bioassay for *in vivo* histamine release effect of GnRH antagonists: prolactin secretion. K. Gordon, R. F. Williams, G. D. Hodgen, USA
22. Inhibitory effect of a highly potent antagonist of LH releasing hormone (SB-75) on the pituitary gonadal axis in the intact and castrated rat. D. Ayalon, Y. Farhi, A. M. Comaru-Schally, A. V. Schally, N. Eckstein, I. Vagman, R. Limor, Israel

2

Mechanism of action of GnRH upon gonadotropin release and synthesis

Z. Naor

Gonadotropin releasing hormone (GnRH) is synthesized in the hypothalamus and released into the hypophyseal portal system in a pulsatile nature to regulate gonadotropin luteinizing hormone (LH) and follicle stimulating hormone (FSH) synthesis and release. GnRH is a member of a family of Ca^{2+} mobilizing ligands which bind to seven transmembrane domain receptors, as indicated recently by the cloning of the GnRH receptor[1,2][27]. The isolated cDNA encodes a 327-amino acid receptor protein with seven putative trans-membrane regions, but lacking the common carboxyl terminal cytoplasmic domain[1,2]. Occupancy of only 20% of GnRH binding sites, located exclusively on pituitary gonadotropes, was sufficient to evoke 80% of the exocytotic response[3]. Since binding affinities were shown to correlate with the biological potencies of various GnRH analogues, it was concluded that the binding sites are indeed receptors[4,5]. GnRH regulates the number of its own receptors in an up- and down-regulation manner, and studies have suggested that protein kinase C is involved in GnRH receptor regulation[4,6,7]. GnRH binds to multi-hormonal gonadotropes (LH + FSH), which constitute about 60% of pituitary gonadotropes, and also to the monohormonal cells (18% LH and 22% FSH cells)[3]. Nevertheless, it is still not clear whether preferential release of LH versus FSH is determined only by the GnRH receptor or, more likely, by a complex interaction and cross-talk of gonadal steroids and peptides (inhibins and activins) with the GnRH receptor[8]. The hormone–receptor complex forms aggregates, and internalization occurs in small vesicles. Exocytosis is manifested when gonadotropin stores in secretory granules are mobilized to specific sites of release. The vesicles may also transfer GnRH to the lysosome for degradation, while multivesicular bodies may be responsible for GnRH receptor recycling. It is not clear yet whether the extrapituitary actions of GnRH analogues are mediated only via GnRH receptors, since direct actions of the GnRH antagonists SB-75 on growth inhibition of breast and endometrial human tumors were attributed to interaction with antagonist receptors, which differ from the GnRH receptors [32].

PHOSPHOINOSITIDE TURNOVER

Following the binding of GnRH to the receptor, a signal transduction cascade is activated by the receptor, which culminates in gonadotropin synthesis and release. Initially, a heterotrimeric guanosine-triphosphate-binding protein (G protein), apparently Gq, is activated[9] [30] (Figure 1). The dissociated α-subunit (αGq) might then activate phospholipase C of the β type in a pertussis-toxin insensitive manner[10,11]. Hydrolysis of phosphatidylinositol-4, 5-bisphosphate (PIP$_2$) by phospholipase C generates inositol-1,4,5-trisphosphate (IP$_3$) and diacylglycerol[12,13]. While IP$_3$ mobilizes intracellular Ca^{2+}, diacylglycerol activates protein kinase C (see references 12–14 for reviews). After a short delay (about 1–2 min), GnRH also activates phospholipase D, as measured by the formation of phosphatidylethanol and phosphatidic acid in the gonadotrope-like cell line αT3-1[15]. Since phosphatidic acid is converted to diacylglycerol by phosphatidic acid phosphohydrolase, it is suggested that diacylglycerol will be provided sequentially by phospholipase C and later by phospholipase D for activation of the various protein kinase C isozymes.

ROLE OF CALCIUM

GnRH requires Ca^{2+} for its action upon gonadotropin secretion. GnRH induces a 'spike-plateau' type of Ca^{2+} mobilization and influx (see reference 14 for review). Internal IP$_3$-sensitive Ca^{2+} pools are responsible for the rapid rise in [Ca^{2+}]$_i$ which is reached a few seconds after stimulation with GnRH. The plateau phase of Ca^{2+} rise is mediated in part by influx of Ca^{2+} through L-type voltage-sensitive and -insensitive Ca^{2+} channels[14]. In single gonadotropes, GnRH induces Ca^{2+} oscillations with dose-dependent modulation of spiking frequency [27]. GnRH also activates apamine-sensitive Ca^{2+}-activated K$^+$ channels, causing episodic waves of plasma membrane hyperpolarization, which seem to be synchronized with the Ca^{2+} transients. The waves of

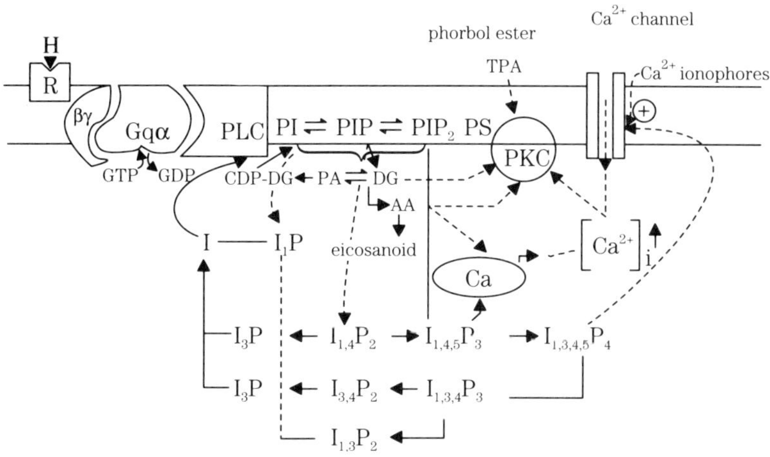

Figure 1 Phosphoinositide turnover. Hormone (H)–receptor (R) interaction results in dissociation of G protein (Gq) and activation of phospholipase C (PLC). PLC hydrolyzes phosphatidylinositol-4, 5-bisphosphate (PIP$_2$) to form diacylglycerol (DG) and inositol-1,4,5-trisphosphate (IP$_3$). DG is then converted to phosphatidic acid (PA) and further to cytosine diphosphate (CDP)-DG which interacts with free inositiol (I) to form phosphatidylinositol (PI). PI is phosphorylated to phosphatidylinositol-4 phosphate (PIP) and back to PIP$_2$. The active isomer of IP$_3$ mobilizes cellular Ca^{2+} pools and is then phosphorylated to IP$_4$. IP$_3$ and IP$_4$ are converted by successive dephosphorylations to inositol (I). DG is also a substrate for DG- and monacylglycerol-lipase whose activation will result in the formation of arachidonic acid (AA) and its metabolites, the eicosanoids

hyperpolarization are also associated with alternating bursts of action potentials which might be involved in Ca^{2+} entry to maintain the IP$_3$ sensitive pools [27]. Gonadal steroids modulate the Ca^{2+} changes induced by GnRH [25]. The importance and mechanisms involved in Ca^{2+} oscillations in general, and in GnRH action in particular, are not known. Interestingly, the profile of GnRH-induced Ca^{2+} mobilization in rat granulosa cells differs from that observed in pituitary cells, since it consists of a transient rise with no sustained phase or oscillations [31]. Pharmacological reconstitution experiments have demonstrated that cellular and extracellular Ca^{2+} is necessary but not sufficient to mediate GnRH-induced gonadotropin secretion (see reference 14 for review). Hence, the search continues for additional messenger molecules involved in GnRH action.

ROLE OF PROTEIN KINASE C

Protein kinase C, a serine/threonine kinase family of related subspecies, plays a major role in cell signalling[13]. The enzyme is involved in synaptic transmission, memory, learning, growth, differentiation, transformation, metabolism, contraction, gene expression and regulation of ion channels. Protein kinase C is also thought to be the main receptor for the tumor promoter phorbol esters. Members of the family consist of conventional types of protein kinase C (α, βI, βII and γ) which are Ca^{2+}/phospholipid dependent, new types of protein kinase C (δ, ϵ, η and θ) and atypical types of protein kinase C (ζ and λ), which are Ca^{2+}-independent, phospholipid-activated enzymes[13]. The co-factors required for protein kinase C activation, Ca^{2+}, diacylglycerol and phosphatidylserine, are generated during phosphoinositide turnover. Diacylglycerol can be produced by phospholipase C and/or phospholipase D, and both are activated by GnRH[10,11,15]. Arachidonic acid, the main product of phospholipase A_2, which can also be produced indirectly by phospholipase C or D, is capable of activating protein kinase βII and protein kinase γ in the absence of the co-factors[16,17]. Pituitary cells express the α, βII, δ, ζ and ϵ subspecies and therefore might be under complex cross-talk of phospholipases C, D and A_2 during protein kinase C activation. Protein kinase C is thought to be activated by translocation to membranes by ligands. Indeed, stimulation with GnRH *in vivo* or *in vitro* resulted in protein kinase C translocation (see reference 14 for review). A major substrate for GnRH was described as a 21-kDa cytosolic protein which can be phosphorylated by GnRH, protein kinases C and A [26]. Depletion of protein kinase C by down-regulation and use of protein kinase C inhibitors have yielded controversial results concerning the role of protein kinase C in GnRH-induced gonadotropin release (see reference 14 for review). Addition of purified activated protein kinase C to protein kinase C-depleted, digitonin-permeabilized pituitary cells showed that, among conventional types of protein kinase C, the α and β, but not γ subspecies stimulated LH release and hence were implicated in GnRH action upon LH release[18]. Protein kinase C was also implicated in GnRH-induced α-subunit and LHβ gene expression[19,20]. Further studies are required to elucidate the role of protein kinase C subspecies in GnRH-induced gonadotropin release and synthesis.

ROLE OF ARACHIDONIC ACID

Arachidonic acid can be liberated from phospholipids by the separate or combined actions of phospholipases C, D and A_2, all of which are thought to be activated by GnRH (see reference 14 for review). It was demonstrated that GnRH increased the formation of the leukotrienes LTC_4, LTD_4 and LTE_4 as well as 5- and 15-eicosatetraenoic acids (HETE)[21,22]. While LTC_4 and LTE_4 enhanced LH release, specific 5-lipoxygenase inhibitors reduced the LH response by 40%. Also, the peptidoleukotriene receptor antagonist ICI 198, 615 inhibited GnRH-induced LH release by 40%. Therefore, a role for arachidonic acid and its lipoxygenase metabolites in GnRH action was suggested[21,22] [24]. The data also suggested a novel amplification cycle in which newly formed leukotrienes become first messengers and establish an autocrine/paracrine loop during the neurohormone action.

GONADOTROPIN BIOSYNTHESIS

The glycoprotein hormones LH, FSH and thyroid stimulating hormone (TSH) share a common α-subunit, but have distinct β-subunits which confer specificity[23]. It is generally agreed that GnRH and gonadal hormones (steroids and peptides) regulate gonadotropin synthesis, but the mechanisms involved are not yet known. The availability of the cDNAs of the gonadotropin subunits and details of the gene structures have opened a new vista of research[23]. Estrogen and cyclic AMP responsive elements have already been described for LH_β, and cAMP responsive elements for the α-subunit. Also, α-gene sequences required for GnRH responsiveness have been found [28]. The effect of GnRH on common α, LH_β and FSH_β mRNA levels was mainly studied *in vivo*. Specific frequencies and the magnitude of GnRH pulses were required to induce optimal stimulation of gonadotropin synthesis. In intact rats desensitized by GnRH, LH_β mRNA levels decreased, while α mRNA levels increased, suggesting that LH_β is tightly coupled to GnRH action [29]. After castration, gonadotropin gene transcription and mRNA levels increased, and decreased after steroid replacement. Steroids were found to have both positive and negative regulation, as well as direct and indirect differential effects on gonadotropin biosynthesis, and their effect can be divergent in different species. The regulation of gonadotropin mRNAs by GnRH *in vitro* is controversial. Some researchers found increased α- but not LH_β mRNA after GnRH stimulus in cells; others found the opposite, and still others found that GnRH increased mRNA levels in both subunits. Recently, a pituitary gonadotrope-like cell line (αT3-1) was derived by targeted tumorigenesis in transgenic mice and is capable of producing the α-subunit[24]. GnRH as well as 12-*O*-tetradecanoyl-phorbol-13-acetate (TPA), forskolin and ionomycin increased α mRNA levels in αT3-1 cells[20,25]. The cell line provides a suitable model to study GnRH action on α-subunit transcription [29]. Further studies are required to elucidate the signal transduction pathways involved in GnRH-induced gonadotropin gene regulation.

CONCLUSIONS

GnRH-induced gonadotropin secretion and synthesis form a multistep process (Figure 2). GnRH binds to a 38-kDa receptor and up- and down-regu-

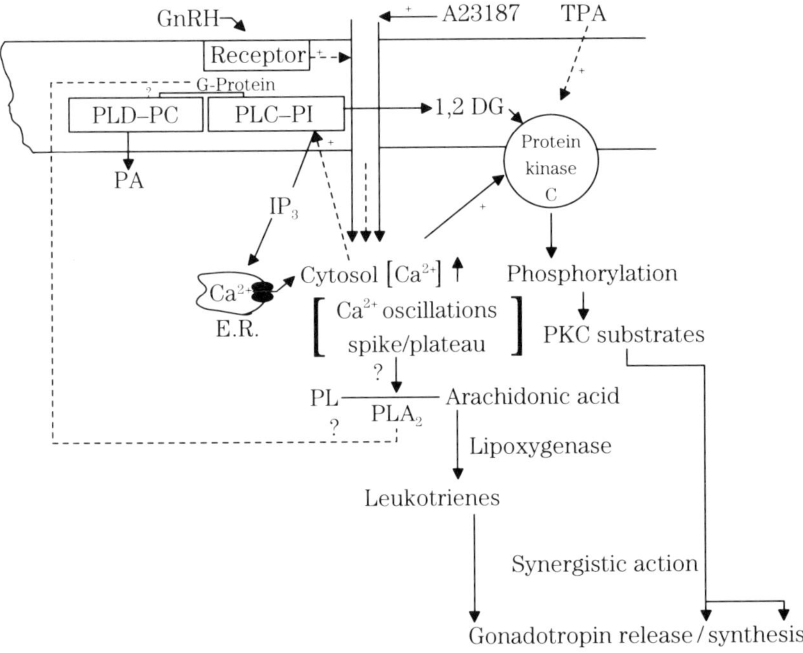

Figure 2 Proposed model for the mechanism of action of GnRH on gonadotropin secretion and gene expression. The activated protein kinase C (PKC) is involved in both release and synthesis. ER, endoplasmic reticulum; PLA2, phospholipase A2; PL, phospholipids; PLD-PC, phosphatidylcholine specific phospholipase D; PLC-PI, phosphatidylinositol specific phospholipase C

lates the number of its own receptors. GnRH activates phospholipase C, most likely by coupling via a GTP-binding protein (Gq).

GnRH also activates phospholipase D activity and furnishes phosphatidic acid, the role of which is still to be determined. Phospholipase C catalyzes a phosphodiesteric hydrolysis of phosphoinositides to form inositol-1,4,5-trisphosphate and diacylglycerol. Inositol-1,4,5-trisphosphate will enhance Ca^{2+} release from intracellular stores[26], which are probably responsible for the first phase of LH release. At the same time, the elevated $[Ca^{2+}]_i$ and diacylglycerol activate protein kinase C which phosphorylates substrate proteins to promote secretion and gonadotropin gene expression. In parallel, $[Ca^{2+}]_i$ is further elevated by Ca^{2+} influx via nifedipine-sensitive and -insensitive channels, which are involved in the second phase of gonadotropin release. Arachidonic acid, which is released at the time of GnRH stimulation, participates also with its lipoxygenase metabolites in gonadotropin exocytosis in an as yet unidentified site. The signaling mechanism involved in GnRH-induced gonadotropin gene expression is as yet unknown.

ACKNOWLEDGEMENTS

The active collaboration of Drs Z. Shraga-Levine, D. Ben-Menahem, N. Reiss, Y. Marantz, R. Rotem, D. Ayalon, I. Hamel, R. Limor and H. Dan-Cohen and Mrs F. Przedecki is greatly appreciated.

The studies were supported by the German–Israeli Foundation for Scientific Research & Development, the United States–Israel Binational Science Foundation, the Israel Cancer Research Fund and the Israel Academy of Sciences & Humanities.

REFERENCES

1. Tsutsumi, M., Zhou, W., Millar, R. P., Mellon, P. L., Roberts, J. L., Flanagan, C. A., Dong, K., Gillo, B. and Sealfon, S. C. (1992). Cloning and functional expression of a mouse gonadotropin-releasing hormone receptor. *Mol. Endocrinol.*, **6**, 1163

2. Reinhart, J., Mertz, L. M. and Catt, K. J. (1992). Molecular cloning and expression of cDNA encoding the murine gonadotropin-releasing hormone receptor. *J. Biol. Chem.*, **267**, 2181

3. Naor, Z. and Childs, G. V. (1986). Binding and activation of gonadotropin releasing hormone receptors in pituitary and gonadal cells. *Int. Rev. Cytol.*, **103**, 147

4. Clayton, R. N. and Catt, K. J. (1981). Gonadotropin releasing hormone receptors: characterization, physiological regulation and relationship to reproductive function. *Endocr. Rev.*, **2**, 186

5. Loumaye, E. and Catt, K. J. (1982). Homologous regulation of gonadotropin-releasing hormone receptors in cultured pituitary cells. *Science*, **215**, 983

6. Naor, Z., Schvartz, I., Hazum, E. and Azrad, A. (1987). Effect of phorbol esters on stimulus–secretion coupling mechanisms in gonadotropin releasing hormone-stimulated pituitary gonadotrophs. *Biochem. Biophys. Res. Commun.*, **148**, 1312

7. Huckle, W. R., McArdle, C. A. and Conn, P. M. (1988). Differential sensitivity of agonist- and antagonist-occupied gonadotropin-releasing hormone receptors to protein kinase C activators. *J. Biol. Chem.*, **263**, 3296

8. Bilezikjian, L. M. and Vale, W. W. (1992). Local extragonadal roles of activins. *Trends Endocrinol. Metab.*, **3**, 218

9. Limor, R., Schvartz, I., Hazum, E., Ayalon, D. and Naor, Z. (1989). Effect of guanine nucleotides as stimulus secretion coupling mechanism in permeabilized pituitary cells: relationship to gonadotropin releasing hormone action. *Biochem. Biophys. Res. Commun.*, **159**, 209

10. Naor, Z., Azrad, A., Limor, R., Zakut, H. and Lotan, M. (1986). Gonadotropin releasing hormone activates a rapid Ca^{2+}-independent phosphodiester hydrolysis of polyphosphoinositides in pituitary gonadotrophs. *J. Biol. Chem.*, **261**, 12506

11. Morgan, R. O., Chang, J. P. and Catt, K. J. (1987). Novel aspects of gonadotropin-releasing hormone action on inositol polyphosphate metabolism in cultured pituitary gonadotrophs. *J. Biol. Chem.*, **262**, 1166

12. Berridge, M. J. (1993). Inositol trisphosphate and calcium signalling. *Nature (London)*, **361**, 315

13. Nishizuka, Y. (1992). Intracellular signaling by hydrolysis of phospholipids and activation of protein kinase C. *Science*, **258**, 607

14. Naor, Z. (1990). Signal transduction mechanisms of Ca^{2+} mobilizing hormones. The case of gonadotropin-releasing hormone. *Endocr. Rev.*, **11**, 326

15. Netiv, E., Liscovitch, M. and Naor, Z. (1991). Delayed activation of phospholipase D by gonadotropin releasing hormone in a clonal pituitary gonadotrope cell line (αT3-1). *FEBS Lett.*, **295**, 107

16. Naor, Z., Shearman, M. S., Kishimoto, A. and Nishizuka, Y. (1988). Calcium-independent activation of hypothalamic type I protein kinase C by *cis*-unsaturated fatty acids. *Mol. Endocrinol.*, **2**, 1043

17. Bell, R. M. and Burns, D. J. (1991). Lipid activation of protein kinase C. *J. Biol. Chem.*, **266**, 4661

18. Naor, Z., Dan-Cohen, H., Hermon, J. and Limor, R. (1989). Induction of exocytosis in permeabilized pituitary cells by α- and β-type protein kinase C. *Proc. Natl. Acad. Sci. USA*, **86**, 450

19. Andrews, W. V., Maurer, R. A. and Conn, P. M. (1980). Stimulation of rat luteinizing hormone-β messenger RNA levels by gonadotropin releasing hormone. *J. Biol. Chem.*, **263**, 13755

20. Ben-Menachem, D., Shraga, Z., Lewy, H., Limor, R., Hammel, I., Stein, R. and Naor, Z. (1992). Dissociation between release and gene expression of gonadotropin α-subunit in GnRH-stimulated αT3-1 cell line. *Biochemistry*, **31**, 12893

21. Kiesel, L., Przylipiak, A. F., Habenicht, A. J. R., Przylipiak, M. S., and Runnebaum, B. (1991). Production of leukotrienes in gonadotropin releasing hormone stimulated pituitary cells. Potential role in luteinizing hormone release. *Proc. Natl. Acad. Sci. USA*, **88**, 8801

22. Dan-Cohen, H., Sofer, Y., Schwartzman, M. L., Natarajan, R. D., Nadler, J. L. and Naor, Z. (1992). GnRH activates the lipoxygenase pathway in cultured pituitary cells. Role in gonadotropin secretion and evidence for a novel autocrine/paracrine loop. *Biochemistry*, **31**, 5442

23. Gharib, S. D., Wierman, M. E., Shupnik, M. A. and Chin, W. W. (1990). Molecular biology of the pituitary gonadotropins. *Endocr. Rev.*, **11**, 177

24. Windle, J. J., Weiner, R. I. and Mellon, P. L. (1990). Cell lines of the pituitary gonadotrope lineage derived by targeted oncogenesis in transgenic mice. *Mol. Endocrinol.*, **4**, 597

25. Horn, F., Bilezikjian, L. M., Perrin, M. H., Bosmat, M. M., Windle, J. J., Huber, K. S., Blount, A. L., Hille, B., Yale, W. W. and Mellon, P. L. (1991). Intracellular responses to gonadotropin releasing hormone in a clonal cell line of the gonadotrope lineage. *Mol. Endocrinol.*, **5**, 347

26. Tse, A., Tse, F. W., Almers, W. and Hille, B. (1993). Rhythmic exocytosis stimulated by GnRH-induced calcium oscillations in rat gonadotropes. *Science*, **260**, 82

BIBLIOGRAPHY

Abstracts of relevant papers presented at the 3rd International Symposium on GnRH Analogues in Cancer and Human Reproduction

24. Intracellular action of gonadotropin-releasing hormone (GnRH) analogues. L. Kiesel, Germany

25. Effects of ovarian steroids on GnRH-induced gonadotropin secretion. G. Emons, K. -D. Schulz, O. Ortmann, Germany

26. GnRH: post-receptor cross-talk between multiple kinase systems in pituitary gonadotropins. T. Makino, S. -I. Izumi, Japan
27. The GnRH receptor: molecular structure and calcium signaling mechanisms. K. J. Catt, J. Reinhart, L. M. Mertz, S. S. Stojilkovic, USA
28. Transcriptional regulation of the α promoter by GnRH. T. W. H. Kay, P. J. Chedrese, S. Pennathur, J. L. Jameson, USA
29. Physiological regulation of gonadotrophin subunit gene expression. R. N. Clayton, UK
30. GnRH receptor-coupled G-protein mediates movement of gonadotropin into a releasable pool: loss of this event is a lesion in the development of homologous desensitization. P. Michael Conn, J. A. Janovick, USA
31. Extra-pituitary actions and signal transaction of GnRH in the ovary and placenta. P. C. K. Leung, Canada
32. A mechanism for direct growth inhibition of human breast and endometrial cancer cells by the GnRH antagonist, SB-75. J. Levy, D. Kleinman, E. Hershkovitz, E. Bosin, T. Segal-Abramson, H. Kitroser, M. Marbach, Y. Sharoni, Israel

3

Application of GnRH analogues in the treatment of female infertility

V. Insler and B. Lunenfeld

A number of gonadotropin releasing hormone (GnRH) analogues (GnRHa), with different amino acid substitutes at position 6 and/or different terminal groups at position 10, are now available for clinical use. Most are marketed in different formulations, presented in various delivery systems and applied at diverse dose levels. Since it is clear that, at least within a certain dose range, the pituitary down-regulation is *not* an all or none phenomenon but its extent and duration are dose-dependent, it is important to recognize the relative effectiveness of each available GnRHa in suppressing pituitary–ovarian function, in order to ascertain well-planned indication-oriented therapy. Van Leusden [1] reviewed the spectrum of biological activity of several GnRHa employed in the treatment of leiomyomata and endometriosis. Since the degree of ovarian suppression required for the former indication is higher than that essential for the latter one, he could pinpoint specific agents particularly appropriate for each treatment.

Filicori and colleagues [4] studied pituitary suppression achieved in normally menstruating women by administration of three consecutive monthly injections of long-acting depot preparations of triptorelin, goserelin or leuprorelin, and compared it to that elicited by daily subcutaneous injections of buserelin applied for similar duration. All analogues used significantly suppressed serum luteinizing hormone (LH) levels by the end of the 3rd month, but the extent of ovarian suppression, as judged by estradiol levels, and pituitary refractoriness as judged by the response to stimulation by native GnRH, were not identical.

37

Coelingh-Bennink and colleagues [2] presented the results of combined treatment regimens using pure recombinant follicle stimulating hormone (FSH) and GnRHa in women undergoing *in vitro* fertilization (IVF). Intranasal buserelin (600 µg daily) in a short and long protocol, and triptorelin in a long protocol with daily subcutaneous injections of 200 µg or a single intramuscular administration of 3.75 µg, were used for pituitary suppression. Ovarian stimulation was performed by administration of recombinant FSH in individually adjusted increasing doses which permitted the achievement of follicles of comparable number and size as well as similar estradiol and FSH levels in all treatment groups on the day of ovulation induction. The LH levels were suppressed in all patients who received GnRHa; they were most profoundly decreased in patients treated with subcutaneous or intramuscular triptorelin. The dose of recombinant FSH required for ovarian stimulation seemed to be negatively correlated with the levels of endogenous LH. The authors concluded that GnRH agonists, irrespective of the type, mode of administration and vehicle used, were incapable to total suppression of LH secretion in cycling women undergoing superovulation induction.

Tarlatzis and his colleagues [3] studied 111 IVF cycles in which the suppression stage was achieved by a long GnRHa protocol, using either intranasal buserelin or subcutaneous leuprolide or intramuscular long-acting triptorelin, and followed by ovarian stimulation with gonadotropins. The incidence of ovarian cysts was 14.8%, 15.3% and 12.9% in the buserelin, leuprolide and triptorelin groups, respectively, the differences between groups not reaching statistical significance.

The conclusions of all the above-cited studies, although very interesting and meaningful, are nevertheless equivocal. On the other hand, it would be of practical importance to know exactly whether certain analogues at certain doses and formulations are particularly suitable for obtaining a specific degree of pituitary and ovarian suppression lasting for a specific period. Such a study, albeit complicated and expensive, should be carried out in the near future, because it would certainly improve our use of certain GnRH analogues at precise doses in distinct clinical situations.

Genazzani and his group [76] studied the serum levels of estradiol, growth hormone, insulin-like growth factor-I (IGF-I), β-endorphin and melanocyte stimulating hormone (MSH) in 12 patients treated with combined GnRHa/ovarian stimulation and in ten women with ovarian stimulation only. No difference in the MSH levels was noted. Estradiol, growth hormone, IGF-I and β-endorphin levels were significantly decreased following pituitary suppression before the stimulation phase. This decrease was offset by subsequent ovarian stimulation. It is possible that the decrease in growth factors and peptides levels is preceded by or connected with hypoestrogenism.

Abnormally high levels of LH during the follicular phase have been shown to exert a detrimental effect upon the follicular development and ovum maturation, resulting in inadequate conception rates and increased pregnancy wastage[1]. Premature LH surges during gonadotropin therapy for induction of superovulation have been blamed for reduced pregnancy rates. Application of GnRHa in the treatment of female infertility has thus been primarily aimed at correcting these two conditions. Indeed, until now the two main indications for employment of GnRHa as adjunctive therapy in ovarian stimulation are controlled ovarian hyperstimulation, usually combined with either *in vitro* fertilization or with intrafallopian gamete (or embryo) transfer or with intrauterine insemination, and polycystic ovarian disease. Obviously, these two topics were extensively discussed at the 3rd International Congress on GnRH Analogues in Cancer and Human Reproduction in 1990.

The general principles of combined pituitary suppression/ovarian stimulation therapy presented several years ago[2] are still relevant (Figure 1). It is

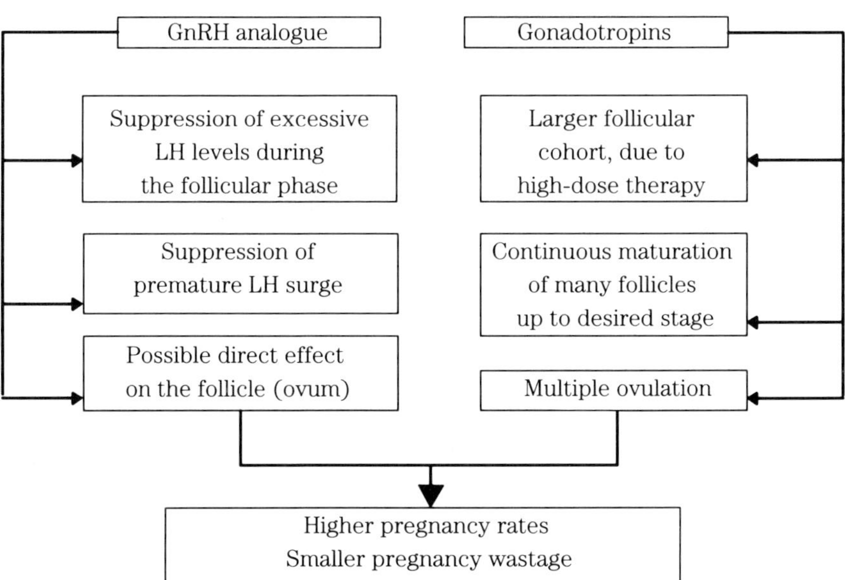

Figure 1 General principles of combined pituitary suppression/ovarian stimulation therapy

important to remember that the combined therapy consists of two distinctive elements: pituitary suppression and ovarian stimulation. Each element exerts specific positive and adverse effects – and only the combination of all the corollaries produces the desired final result.

The general tenor of the sessions dealing with assisted reproduction techniques has been that pituitary suppression by GnRHa as an adjunctive therapy to controlled ovarian hyperstimulation significantly improves the overall results of assisted reproduction techniques. Since the best indicator of efficacy of any infertility treatment is the 'take home baby' rate, the reports of Tan and his colleagues [80] and of Braendle and his colleagues [79] are of particular interest. Tan's group analyzed data pertaining to 7863 consecutive IVF cycles in 4115 women, resulting in 1279 clinical pregnancies and 764 live births. The cumulative live birth rate has been significantly higher in cycles treated with combined pituitary suppression by GnRHa and ovarian stimulation by gonadotropins with or without clomiphene citrate than in cycles treated by ovarian stimulation only. The cumulative live birth rate after three cycles was 55% in the former group and 34% in the latter group, respectively. Multiple logistic regression analysis indicated that the odds of having a live birth with combined therapy, as compared to stimulation treatment, adjusted for age, cause of infertility, attempt number and year of treatment, was 1.97.

Braendle's group assessed the course and outcome of 179 pregnancies after combined GnRHa/human menopausal gonadotropin (hMG) therapy and 66 pregnancies following gonadotropin treatment only [79]. The abortion rate was slightly higher after combined GnRHa/hMG therapy (20%) as compared to hMG treatment (14.0%). The rates of tubal pregnancies and multiple gestations were similar in the two groups (2.8% and 3%, 22% and 26%, respectively). The birth weight was different between single, twin and triplet pregnancies, but was not dependent on the stimulation protocol used. This study indicates that pituitary suppression preceding ovarian stimulation does not adversely influence the course and outcome of pregnancy, thus accentuating the advantages of this therapy, such as lower cancellation rate, patients' comfort, and organizational and planning improvement.

Nafarelin, a GnRHa characterized by substitution of the original amino acid at position 6 by D2-naphtyl-alanine, has been recently introduced into wide clinical trials. The results of these endeavors were extensively discussed by Lockwood and colleagues [69], Lopes and colleagues [70], Alvarez and co-workers [71] and Yuzpe and his colleagues [72]. Doses of 400, 600 and 800 µg per day were employed intranasally. All authors agree that nafarelin

Table 1   Effect of different GnRH analogues on results of *in vitro* fertilization

Reference	Number of cycles	Agonist	Dose	Route of application	Results Pregnancy/ET (%)
[69]	240	buserelin	200 µg × 5	i.n.	39.1
		nafarelin	200 µg b.i.d	i.n.	36.7
		nafarelin	400 µg b.i.d.	i.n.	39.1
[70]	38	nafarelin	200 µg b.i.d.	i.n.	41.7
		triptorelin	0.1 mg/day	s.c.	8.3
[71]	277	buserelin	300 µg b.i.d.	i.n.	overall
		nafarelin	200 µg b.i.d.	i.n.	28.0
		nafarelin	400 µg b.i.d.	i.n.	
[72]	379	leuprolide	0.5 mg/day	s.c.	overall
		nafarelin	200 µg b.i.d.	i.n.	similar
		nafarelin	200 µg t.i.d.	i.n.	
[77]	31	goserelin	3.6 mg	i.m.	37.0
[73]	25 421	triptorelin	3.75 mg	i.m.	Delivery/OPU IVF 12% GIFT 20%

i.n., intranasal; s.c., subcutaneous; i.m., intramuscular;, OPU, ovum pick-up; IVF, *in vitro* fertilization; GIFT, gamete intrafallopian transfer

at a daily dose of 800 µg is equally effective as subcutaneous leuprolide and as intranasal buserelin in the framework of *in vitro* fertilization–embryo transfer (IVF–ET), gamete intrafallopian transfer (GIFT) or zygote intrafallopian transfer (ZIFT) programs (Table 1). There are not enough data to determine whether the low dosage (200 µg b.i.d.) is equally effective.

The results obtained with a single injection of long-acting GnRHa were also reported. Germer and his colleagues [77] treated 31 hyperandrogenic patients with combined goserelin 3.6 mg/hMG therapy and Zorn and co-workers [73] reported the results of 25 421 IVF–ET or GIFT cycles in two-thirds of which (approximately 17 000) a combination of decapeptyl LP 3.75 mg with gonadotropins was used. They concluded that a single injection of a long-acting GnRHa:

(1) Is adequate for pituitary suppression;

(2) Is more comfortable for the patients;

(3) Enables the planning of the work of IVF clinic to be arranged several months in advance;

(4) Ensures that the persistence of minimal amounts of GnRHa at the time of implantation has no adverse effect on the pregnancy rate and fetal well-being.

Whether inadvertent application of GnRHa at conception or during the implantation period or in early pregnancy has an effect on the offspring has yet to be proven. Some animal experiments seem to indicate a possible adverse effect on testicular function in male offspring. Some cases of small-for-gestational-age babies, cleft palate and some other minor malformations were reported in humans. Roux and colleagues [137], on the other hand, reviewed 20 patients who were inadvertently administered triptorelin (Decapeptyl®, Ferring) between the 1st and 4th month of gestation. Eighteen patients delivered normal babies with an average weight of 3225 kg.

The effectiveness of long, short and ultrashort protocols for pituitary suppression in the framework of assisted reproduction techniques was discussed by Chang and colleagues [75], Tarlatzis and colleagues [82], Torok and colleagues [83] and Tzeng and colleagues [84] (Table 2). Definitive analysis of the data presented is not possible because various authors used different end-points in their study protocols. In general, however, these presentations clearly indicate that, so far as pregnancy rates in IVF or GIFT programs are regarded, the long protocol is more effective than the short and ultrashort

Table 2   Comparison of effects of long and short protocols for pituitary suppression with GnRH analogues in assisted reproduction cycles

			Results	
Reference	*Number of cycles*	*Protocol*	*Pregnancies per ET*	*Implantation rate*
[75]	NS	long	37.2%	
	NS	ultrashort	37.6%	
[82]	192	long		15.3
	116	short		9.3
[83]	NS	long	higher	
	NS	short	lower	
[84]	73	ultrashort	33.0%	

NS, not stated

ones. Our own experience and several recent publications also support this conclusion.

Tan and his co-workers [81] were also able to show that the long pituitary suppression protocol provided an ovulation induction window of at least 3 days' duration during which human chorionic gonadotropin (hCG) can be administered with equally good results. This might enable simplification of monitoring of IVF cycles to an absolute minimum, reducing the cost and increasing patients' comfort.

Hopes were raised as to the possible use of GnRHa for induction of ovulation in women with premature ovarian failure. The rationale of this suggestion was that lack of ovarian response to exogenous stimulation in these women was due to both ovarian insensitivity and abnormally high gonadotropin levels. Van Kasteren and co-workers [74] report on a prospective double-blind placebo-controlled randomized study in 30 women suffering from premature ovarian failure. The study protocol consisted of four phases:

(1) No treatment for 4 weeks;

(2) Either buserelin 1 mg daily or placebo intranasally for 3 weeks;

(3) In addition to the medication of phase 2, increasing doses of FSH (starting with 150 IU and ending with 450 IU daily) were added;

(4) No treatment during 4 weeks.

Follicular development was judged by ultrasonography and urinary estrogen levels. Whenever the largest follicle exceeded 18 mm in diameter and/or the urinary estrogen level was higher than 500 nmol/l, hCG was administered for ovulation induction. Follicular development occurred in 5/15 patients receiving buserelin and in 4/15 women in the placebo group. The ovulation rate in the buserelin group (20%) was not significantly different from the placebo group (0%). The authors conclude that addition of GnRH agonist to the ovulation induction regimen is not beneficial for the treatment results in women with premature ovarian failure.

Polycystic ovarian disease is one of the most controversial, interesting and challenging gynecological entities. A considerable proportion of women suffering from ovulation disturbances and/or repeated pregnancy wastage are eventually diagnosed as having polycystic ovaries. Standard clomiphene therapy has been believed to bring about a conception rate of approximately 30%, and hMG treatment could be expected to yield some additional 25% of pregnancies in this group of patients. Although there is quite a discrepancy between the actual numbers, all authors agree that in patients with polycystic ovarian disease treatment-induced gestations are prone to end at the chemical pregnancy stage, in the pre-implantation period or in the first trimester, and that, consequently, the 'take-home-baby' rate is dramatically lower than in other groups of infertile women. Based on animal experiments and clinical experience, a concept was formulated associating abnormally high LH levels during the follicular phase of the cycle with 'premature aging of ova' which, in turn, could be the reason for anovulation or lack of conception or pregnancy wastage. To overcome the 'LH obstacle', some authors advocated the induction of ovulation in patients with polycystic ovarian disease with 'pure' FSH rather than with hMG containing equal amounts of both FSH and LH, and claimed that the former produced significantly better results than the latter. However, many groups were unable to confirm these findings. Treatment combining gonadotropin suppression by GnRHa and ovarian stimulation by exogenous FSH seemed to be a more favorable proposition. Indeed, this was amply emphasized in presentations during this Congress.

Birkhauser and his co-workers [86] summarized the results of therapy in 57 infertile women suffering from clomiphene-resistant hyperandrogenic anovulation. Application of FSH alone in 131 cycles resulted in a success rate of 57%. Those patients who did not respond to the FSH therapy because of premature LH surges were subsequently treated with a combination of intranasal buserelin (900 µg daily) and intramuscular injections of purified FSH. The combined regimen yielded a pregnancy rate of 65%, and the cumulative success rate in this group of 57 women treated by FSH alone and selectively by combined therapy was 74%.

Collins [87] used combined leuprolide/hMG therapy in 39 women with polycystic ovarian disease who previously had failed to conceive when treated with either clomiphene citrate or hMG. The suppression/stimulation regimen resulted in a conception rate of 72%.

Homburg and his group [88] analyzed treatment results in a rather sizable group of 239 women with polycystic ovarian disease who had all failed to respond to clomiphene therapy. A total of 110 patients received combined GnRHa/hMG treatment and 129 hMG therapy alone. In both groups, ovulation was induced by hCG. Co-treatment with GnRHa mildly improved the cumulative conception rate but significantly enhanced the cumulative live birth rate (64% in the combined treatment and 26% in the hMG alone therapy, respectively).

The study of Hompes and colleagues [89] supports the theory of the deleterious effect of abnormally high LH levels on follicular development. They treated 12 patients with polycystic ovarian disease with pulsatile GnRH, either directly or after a 3-week pretreatment with GnRHa. The levels of LH during the 12 days before ovulation were significantly lower in the latter group. The conception rates were similar in both groups, but the ongoing pregnancy rate was better in patients pretreated with GnRHa as compared to those who received pulsatile therapy alone.

Fauser proposed a step-down combined therapy in which, after achieving pituitary suppression by GnRHa, FSH was administered in successively decreasing doses. He claimed that this treatment produced a more uniform follicular cohort and, consequently, acceptable ovulation rates with lower incidence of multiple ovulations and ovarian hyperstimulation syndrome. This concept is certainly interesting and, if adopted and tested by other groups, may turn out to be an original treatment regime for polycystic ovarian disease. It seems that, at present, the treatment of infertility in women with polycystic ovarian disease should conform to the algorithm based on the initial response to clomiphene (Figure 2).

Some authors pointed out that polycystic ovarian disease becomes fully expressed at or around puberty. They suggested that diagnosis at this time and preventive therapy could perhaps delay the onset of symptomatology or diminish the full development of the disease or reduce the severity of complications. In this context, the study of Nizzoli and his colleagues [90] is of particular interest. They described four young girls with clinical, hormonal and sonographic diagnosis of polycystic ovarian disease who have been continuously treated with monthly injections of a long-acting GnRHa. This therapy caused a significant decrease in ovarian volume and a normalization of gonadotropin and steroid profiles in all patients. However, in one girl who interrupted therapy after 1 year, a reappearance of sonographic and hormonal features of the disease was observed within 3 months. This indicates that prolonged pituitary suppression may reduce the severity of signs and symptoms but is most probably not capable of removing the cause of the disease.

Presentations and discussions at the 3rd International Congress on GnRH Analogues in Cancer and Human Reproduction have shown once more that GnRHa, as an adjunctive regimen in the induction of ovulation and superovulation in infertile women, are here to stay. In polycystic ovarian disease, this therapy significantly improves the 'take-home-baby' rate, and in induction of

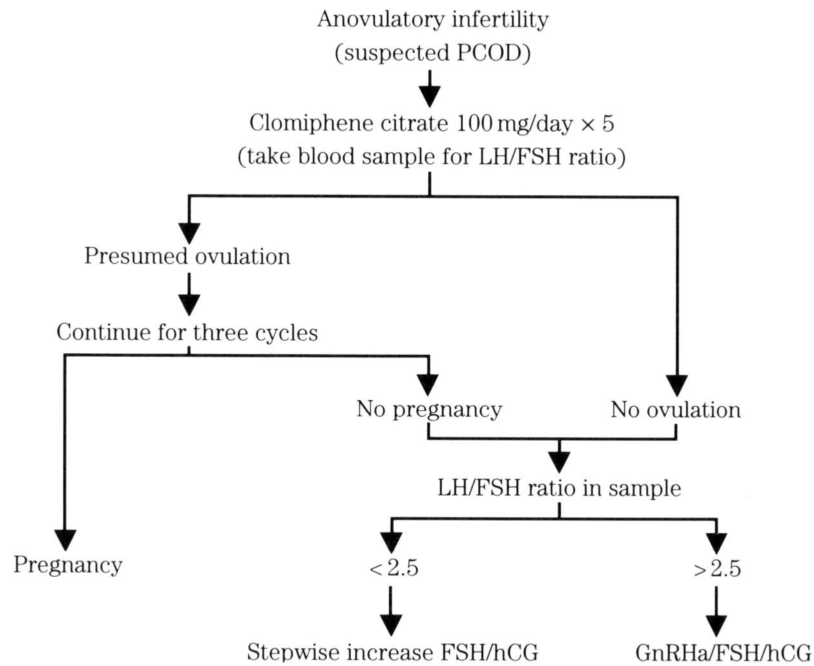

Figure 2 Proposed algorithm for ovulation induction in infertile patients with polycystic ovarian disease (PCOD). Blood sample for LH estimation should be taken 1–3 days after cessation of clomiphene

superovulation it improves the organization of treatment, reduces the cancellation rate, amplifies patients' comfort and augments conception rates by allowing more intense ovarian stimulation by gonadotropins.

REFERENCES

1. Shoham, Z., Jacobs, H. S. and Insler, V. (1993). Luteinizing hormone: its role, mechanism of action and detrimental effects when hypersecreted during the follicular phase. *Fertil. Steril.*, in press
2. Insler, V., Lunenfeld, B., Potashnik, G. and Levy, J. (1990). The combined pituitary suppression/ovarian stimulation therapy: myths and realities. In Mashiach, S., Ben-Rafael, Z., Laufer, N. and Schenker, J. G. (eds.) *Advances in Assisted Reproductive Technologies*, pp. 31–8. (New York: Plenum Press)

BIBLIOGRAPHY

Abstracts of relevant papers presented at the 3rd International Symposium on GnRH Analogues in Cancer and Human Reproduction

1. Clinical impact of different analogues, due to their chemical nature and delivery systems in benign gynecology. H.A.I.M. Van Leusden, The Netherlands
2. GnRH agonists are incapable of total suppression of LH in ovarian superovulation for IVF. H. Coelingh-Bennink, B. Mannaerts, A. van Steirteghem, P. Devroey, Belgium
3. Follicle cyst formation after administration of different GnRH analogues for assisted reproduction. B. C. Tarlatzis, H. Bili, J. Bontis, S. Lagos, S. Mantalenakis, Greece
4. Effects of different depot GnRH analogs on pituitary and ovarian function in women. M. Filicor, G. Cognigni, P. Dellai, A. Falbo, Italy
69. A prospective randomized single-blind comparative trial of nafarelin acetate with buserelin in long protocol GnRH analogue controlled IVF treatments. G. M. Lockwood, D. H. Barlow, UK
70. A randomised comparison of nafarelin nasal spray and triptorelin s.c. in a short protocol of stimulation prior to IVF. P. Lopes, P. Barriere, V. Julou, M. F. Dubin, M. Benelli, M. Jean, L. Ory-Lavollee, France
71. A randomised multicenter comparison between nafarelin nasal spray and buserelin sc for down-regulation prior to ovarian stimulation in an IVF program. S. Alvarez, C. Lelandier, A. Cataneo, B. Hedon, R. Frydman, J. Salat-Baroux, L. Ory-Lavollee, France
72. A comparison between two doses of nafarelin acetate and leuprolide for pituitary down-regulation in *in vitro* fertilization. A. A. Yuzpe, E. Yuzpe, B. Kaplan, J. Nisker, I. Tummon, S. Daniel, Canada
73. Efficiency and safety of the long lasting preparation decapeptyl, 3,75 LP, for ovarian stimulation in IVF–ET cycles. J. R. Zorn, M. El Sadek, K. Terras, B. Schatz, G. Caillaud, France
74. Ovulation induction in patients with premature ovarian failure (POF) after pituitary desensitization: a placebo-controlled double-blind randomized trial. Y. M. van Kasteren, A. Hoek, P. G. A. Hompes, J. Schoemaker, The Netherlands
75. Use of GnRH agonist in IVF program. Y. S. Chang, J. Y. Lee, S. H. Kim, Korea
76. Clinical use of GnRH analogue in induction of superovulation: effects on growth factors and peptides. A. R. Genazzani, C. Battaglia, F. Droghini, G. G. Umoh, G. D'Ambrogio, P. G. Artini, Italy
77. Goserelin/hMG stimulation for *in vitro* fertilisation in hyperandrogenic patients. U. Germer, R. K. Schmutzler, K. Diedrich, C. Diedrich, D. Dumont, Dos Santos, C. Tunnermann, S. AlHasani, D. Krebs, Germany

the staging classification of endometriosis when associated with infertility and the condition as it affects patients with no infertility problems. Also included in this new classification will be the incorporation of the morphological activity of the endometrial implants. It is proposed that these staging classifications be validated before they are published.

With respect to treatment, endometriosis may be managed medically or by surgical approach. Severe endometriosis consistent with late AFS III or IV stages should be treated primarily by surgery. Surgical management may be supplemented with pre- and/or postoperative medical therapy, as deemed appropriate.

In most centers, endometriotic lesions are initially treated by laser ablation, fulgurization or excision at the time of diagnostic laparoscopy. Thereafter, symptomatic disease is commonly treated with medication.

What are the options? Combination oral contraceptives, pure progestogens, danazol and gonadotropin releasing hormone (GnRH) analogues all seem to be effective but are associated with different side-effects and patient tolerance[1,2].

The eight papers presented in the symposium devoted to endometriosis [61–68] concentrated on hormonal management of this disease.

Crosignani [61] reviewed all of the papers published in the English literature between 1970 and 1991 on the use of medroxyprogesterone acetate (MPA), gestrinone, danazol and GnRH agonist in the treatment of pelvic pain in patients with endometriosis. He identified a total of three studies on MPA, four on gestrinone, 13 on danazol and 17 on GnRH agonists. Most of these studies were non-comparative open trials. Considered together, these studies indicated that the frequency of pelvic pain at the end of treatment (non-responders) was 3% for women treated with MPA, 6% for those treated with gestrinone, 17% for those treated with danazol and 11% for patients receiving GnRH agonists. These differences were not statistically significant. These data suggest that the efficacy of MPA, gestrinone, danazol and GnRH agonists in the treatment of pelvic pain for endometriosis are largely comparable. However, despite favorable results during treatment, about 50% of women experienced recurrence of pelvic pain a few months following the termination of treatment.

Schindler and associates [62] presented the results of a multicenter study using buserelin intranasally in a dose of 900 μg/day, for the management of endometriosis in five German universities. The study involved 452 patients who received the agonist for a period of 6 months. The relief of endometriosis and the decrease in AFS classification staging of the disease, as well as the incidence of various side-effects, were similar to studies reported previously with other agonists. This large clinical study demonstrated, once again, the effectiveness of a GnRH agonist for the reduction of endometriotic lesions and improvement of clinical symptoms. A similar study involving 60 patients and comparing triptorelin versus danazol was reported by Ochs and colleagues [66].

The concept of add-back therapy using a GnRH agonist with the addition of an estrogen or estrogen/progestogen combination has recently received considerable attention. It is argued that the GnRH agonist threshold for suppression of endometriotic lesions and relief of symptoms may be different from that of bone mineral loss. Thus, the addition of a small dose of estrogen and/or progestogen may alleviate some of the hypoestrogenic effects of GnRH agonists while preserving their effectiveness. The paper of Geisthovel [63] addressed this issue. He studied eight patients suffering from recurrent endometriosis stages III and IV (AFS classification) with monthly injections of triptorelin combined with an estrogen/progestogen replacement therapy (Cycloprogynova®, Schering). He observed relief of symptoms without the occurrence of side-effects. Another randomized controlled study, combining subcutaneous goserelin 3.6 mg once a month and MPA 100 mg/day orally versus goserelin plus placebo, was reported by Kauppila and colleagues [64]. Twenty-seven patients received GnRH analogue plus MPA and 24 received GnRH analogue and placebo. At the end of 6 months of treatment, the results indicated that both regimens caused a similar decrease in the size of endometriotic lesions and relief of symptoms. Additionally, the patients with added MPA menstruated sooner (60 days) compared to those receiving placebo (75 days) following the discontinuation of therapy. Kauppila's group also reported the important finding that MPA did not antagonize the suppressive action of GnRH analogue on endometriotic lesions, as reported previously[3]. Fedele and associates [68] performed structural and ultrastructural studies of the vaginal mucosa in women receiving GnRH agonist or danazol for a period of 3 months. Buserelin treatment induced early, marked hypotrophy of the vaginal mucosa with features similar to that of the menopause. The modifications caused by danazol were lighter and occurred mainly in the intermediate layer, which was weakly hypotrophic.

Collectively, these studies confirm previous reports that various GnRH agonists are potent therapeutic agents for the management of endometriosis and bring about not only the suppression of endometrial lesions but also relief of symptoms. These results are generally comparable to those using danazol and progestational agents.

A novel aspect of treatment with GnRH agonist regimens is the addition of estrogen and/or progestogen to alleviate hypoestrogenic symptoms and to prevent the loss of bone mineral content. Preliminary results from this symposium and a small series of cases reported elsewhere indicate that, in fact, the add-back regimen may accomplish these goals. Admittedly, larger controlled multicenter studies currently in progress are required effectively to prove these concepts.

How should the average physician, not involved in research or drug evaluation, treat endometriosis? What are his options and which is the drug of choice? The selection of the drug of choice is based on several factors including effectiveness, response of the patient, side-effects and last, but not the least, the cost.

Assuming equal effectiveness between progestogens and danazol and available GnRH agonists, as has been reported, the deciding factor in selecting a drug will be based on the degree of the patient's tolerance, lack of major side-effects and the cost. Because of the chronic nature of endometriosis, the average symptomatic patient will probably require and receive several courses of medical therapy during her reproductive life. Some women will unquestionably exhibit side-effects to one or several of these drugs, others will be unresponsive or intolerant. The availability of several drugs enables the physician to select the most suitable medication for the patient at any given time.

REFERENCES

1. Moghissi, K. S. (1992). Office management of endometriosis. In: Stenchever, M. (ed.), pp. 413–29. *Office Gynecology*, (St. Louis: Mosby-Yearbook)
2. Moghissi, K. S. (1990). Gonadotropin releasing hormones. Clinical applications in gynecology. *J. Reprod. Med.*, **35**, 1097–107
3. Cedars, M. I., Lu, J. K. H., Meldrum, D. R. and Judd, H. L., (1990). Treatment of endometriosis with a long acting gonadotropin releasing hormone agonist plus medroxyprogesterone acetate. *Obstet. Gynecol.*, **75**, 641

BIBLIOGRAPHY

Abstracts of relevant papers presented at the 3rd International Symposium on GnRH Analogues in Cancer and Human Reproduction

61. The efficacy of medroxyprogesterone acetate, gestrinone, danazol and gonadotrophin releasing hormone agonist in the treatment of pelvic pain for endometriosis: a quantitate review of the literature. P. G. Crosignani, Italy

62. Treatment of endometriosis with the GnRH-agonist buserelin: a multicenter study. A. E. Schindler, K. Buhler, L. Mettler, U. Fuchs, U. Cirkel, H. Ochs, K. -W. Schweppe, R. Koch, Germany

63. GnRII-analogue plus estrogen/gestagen replacement therapy: an alternative treatment of severe recurrent endometriosis. F. Geisthovel, Germany

64. Treatment of endometriosis with GnRH agonist analog supplemented with progestin. A placebo-controlled trial. A. Kauppila, L. Makarainen, L. Ronnberg, Finland

65. GnRH analogue depot (Triptorelin) versus danazol in the treatment of endometriosis. U. Cirkel, H. Ochs, P. G. Schneider, Germany

66. Correlation between extent of ovarian suppression and regression of endometriosis: Decapeptyl vs danazol. H. Ochs, U. Cirkel, H. P. G. Schneider, Germany

67. Treatment of endometriosis with GnRH agonist leuprorelin acetate depot (Enantone-Gyn). A multicenter study. A. E. Schindler, Germany

68. Three months therapy for endometriosis with a GnRH agonist and danazol: structural and ultrastructural aspects of vaginal mucosa. I. Fedele, M. Marchini, S. Bianchi, L. Tozzi, R. Mezzopane, F. Zanotti, Italy

5

GnRH analogues in the management of uterine leiomyomas and other benign gynecological situations

G. Benagiano, F. M. Primiero and C. Villani

Leaving aside endometriosis, which has been dealt with separately, the pharmacological treatment of uterine leiomyomata – either as an adjunct, or as a substitute to surgical management – still represents the most important gynecological application of GnRH analogues (GnRHa). There are, however, a number of other, probably less frequent, although not necessarily less important, clinical applications of this class of compounds.

A number of such new indications have been discussed during the Third International Symposium on GnRH Analogues in Cancer and Human Reproduction. They include both gynecological and non-gynecological conditions; in both cases, analogues are utilized to obtain a positive effect on the female reproductive tract.

It is the purpose of this paper to review and summarize the place of GnRHa in the management of uterine fibroids, as well as other indications, in the light of experience accumulated over the last decade.

UTERINE FIBROIDS

Treatment is, logically, the last link in the chain of events leading to the successful management of an illness. Successful therapy, therefore, presupposes appropriate knowledge of the origin, natural history and factors influencing the course of any disease. This knowledge, in the case of uterine leiomyomas, has been inadequate and it is only in the last decade or so that

55

a variety of investigations have attempted to elucidate their genesis and the role of the hormonal milieu in their growth.

This new information has had a great influence in opening the way to new therapeutic modalities, which will eventually revolutionize the exclusively surgical treatment of these benign tumors.

Pathophysiology

Uterine leiomyomas are the most common form of pathological growth in the female reproductive tract; even before the advent of modern imaging technology, it was estimated that they occur in some 25% of all women[1]. Routine ultrasound scanning has confirmed the presence, during the reproductive years, of small, asymptomatic fibroid masses in many otherwise normal uteri. Leiomyomas are most frequently observed in women in their fifth decade and, if menopause is delayed until after 50 years, they may affect almost 40% of all women[2]. They are between three and nine times more frequent in Negroid than in Caucasian women[3,4]; this higher occurrence may be due to more frequent pelvic infection with an ensuing myometrial irritation[5].

Several risk factors for fibroids have been identified: nulliparity, unopposed estradiol production due to anovulation, obesity[6]. In addition, isolated reports published in the 1970s suggested that oral contraceptive pills may promote myoma growth[7]. Large epidemiological studies, however, have clearly shown that oral contraceptive use for 10 years decreases by more than 30% the risk of developing fibroids; the risk is also decreased among women who smoke[6].

Histogenesis

The origin of leiomyomas remains obscure, although theories on their histogenesis date back to the last century. Virchow believed that myomas could be generated by each muscle cell of the uterus[8], a view more recently substantiated by the finding that cells constituting a tumor contain the same electrophoretic type of glucose-6-phosphate dehydrogenase and that the type of the enzyme may vary among different fibroids within the same uterus[9]. Opitz, on the other hand, believed that they do not arise from muscle cells but from the surrounding connective tissue and claimed to have traced, in serial sections of small myomas, the gradual metaplasia from one cell to the other[8]. Several authors supposed the existence of indifferent embryonic[10], primitive mesenchymal[5], or even immature[11,12] muscle cells that, when properly stimulated, would develop into leiomyomas. One theory holds that they spring from the adventitia and media of vascular walls[8], or from muscle cells in their proximity[13].

More recent investigations have demonstrated the presence of clonal chromosomal aberrations in some myoma cells[14]. A number of anomalies have been recently described. Translocation and rearrangement of chromosomes 12 and 14 may be specifically associated with these tumors[15–18], although a chromosome 7 deletion has been observed, isolated[19] or in association[20], and, in all published series, apparently normal karyotypes are also present.

Deichert and colleagues [50] administered goserelin to 14 women harboring fibroids and, following surgery, studied the karyotype of myomatous cells: in two cases the cell culture failed; in nine the karyotype was normal, whereas various clonal aberrations were observed in the last three.

The often positive family history in patients suffering from leiomyomas ('fibroids run in families'[8]) led to the suggestion of the presence of a gene encoding for fibroid development[21].

The role of the hormonal milieu

Whatever their origin, it is clear that the growth of leiomyomas is greatly influenced by the hormonal milieu. This fact was recognized long before steroid hormones were identified: Lockyer, in his informative book on myomas published in 1918[8], reports to have performed oophorectomy to stop the growth and reduce the size of a large fibroid tumor. Many facts support the theory that estrogens influence the growth of leiomyomas: they are exceptional before puberty[7,22,23], are most frequent after 40 years of age[2,23] when estrogen production is usually unopposed, and regress after menopause[24].

Fibromas contain estrogen receptors, although it is controversial whether their concentration is higher in tumor tissue[25–33]. Two types of estrogen receptors have been isolated: type I have high affinity, low capacity and bind estradiol by competitive binding. Type II, on the contrary, have low affinity, high capacity and bind estradiol by positive cooperation[34]. Recently Otsuka and colleagues[35], in a careful comparative evaluation, confirmed that estrogen receptor content in myomas tends to be higher than in normal myometrium, although the difference was not significant. When, however, they determined by immunocytochemistry the pattern of distribution of estrogen receptors, the concentration per cell was statistically significantly higher in tumor tissue, suggesting that leiomyomas contain more estrogen receptor-positive cells. Maximum receptor induction is reached between days 10 and 18 of the cycle, at the time when estrogen production is highest[32].

Cirkel and colleagues [38] compared receptors in six uteri removed during the follicular phase of untreated women with symptomatic myomas and those in 14 myomas enucleated after 6 months of leuprolide treatment. In untreated subjects, there was a predominance of receptor-positive cells in the basal cell layer of the cervix. The frequency of estrogen receptor-positive cells decreased in the endometrium; in contradistinction to this, progesterone-positive staining was abundantly present. The action of GnRHa resulted in a decrease in the estrogen receptor content, but not in progesterone receptors.

In spite of an abundance of data suggesting a close relationship between estrogens and the induction and/or growth of leiomyomas, the mechanism of action of the hormone is still unclear. The levels of estradiol[36,37], progesterone, FSH and LH[37] in women harboring fibroids do not differ from normal controls. This, however, does not exclude a tumor-selective higher sensitivity to estrogens, or a local higher production in or around the myomatous tissue. Several facts support the latter hypothesis: submucous fibromas are surrounded by a limited zone of endometrial glandular hyperplasia[38,39], and estrone sulfatase activity, as well as estrone concentration, are higher in the endometrium overlying leiomyomas[40]. These data suggest that the milieu surrounding the tumor is hyperestrogenic. In addition, conversion of estradiol into estrone is significantly lower in tumor tissue[41]; this, in turn, is reflected by a relatively low concentration of estrone[40] and a very high one of estradiol[42].

Another important parameter to consider, in evaluating factors influencing the growth of myomas, is the role played by progesterone. It is well documented that leiomyomas contain progesterone receptors[42–46]. Receptor concentration seems higher in the tumor[44] and decreases both after administration of estrogens and progestins[43–45]. The effect of GnRH superagonist analogue (GnRHa) therapy is controversial[33,42]. Against this background, interactions between estradiol and progesterone in fibroid tissue seem complex: in pregnancy, leiomyomas tend to grow during the first half[47], but usually regress later on, occasionally showing the so-called red degeneration[48]. The addition of a progestogen to GnRHa therapy greatly decreases its effectiveness[49], whereas, if the progestin is administered after analogues have produced their effect, it can prevent tumor regrowth[50].

It has been speculated that the growth of leiomyomas during pregnancy may be caused by a synergistic effect of estradiol and human placental lactogen (hPL), which is biologically similar to growth hormone[51], although the role of the latter in the pathogenesis of leiomyomas is not clear, and it is difficult to explain the degenerative changes occurring during the second part of a pregnancy when hPL and estrogen levels are highest.

Another factor probably involved in the growth of myomas is epidermal growth factor (EGF), first identified in fibroid tissue in 1984[52]; EGF binds to a lower extent to tumor cells than to normal myometrium[53], and this binding capacity is decreased even further if hypoestrogenism occurs[33,54]. Finally, the platelet-derived growth factor, for which more receptor sites exist in myomas, can be considered, with insulin, as an additional potential regulator of uterine fibroid growth[53].

Leiomyoma extracts contain mitogen(s) which stimulate cells with fibroblast, myoblast and osteoblast phenotype. This activity is absent in normal myometrial extracts and may play a role in the dynamics of the tumor[55].

An interesting observation, that may be relevant to studies of the mechanism of action of GnRHa on leiomyomas, is that they contain specific binding sites for GnRH[56].

Johannisson and colleagues [51] evaluated the DNA synthesis in leiomyoma cells separated by collagenase, before and after treatment with decapeptyl: 3 months of treatment significantly decreased the proliferative activity of the fibroma cells assessed by DNA analysis ($p = 0.001$).

Malignant degeneration

Malignant degeneration of leiomyomas is very rare, since it is estimated that leiomyosarcomas occur in 0.67 per 100 000 women[57]. Indeed, unexpected sarcomatous degeneration occurred in 0.17%[58] and 0.49%[59], respectively in two large series of surgical myoma specimens. Since malignant degeneration occurs more often in postmenopausal patients[60–62], it does not seem to pose a significant threat in younger women.

Notwithstanding these reassuring epidemiological data, a number of reports have indicated the occurrence of a case of leiomyosarcoma in a relatively small series of women treated with analogues for uterine fibroids[63,64] [55]. Therefore, its possible occurrence must be kept in mind in the event of rapid growth not blocked by GnRHa therapy. The principal features of leiomyosarcomas observed in connection with GnRHa treatment are:

(1) Age: the fifth or sixth decade of life;

(2) Appearance: an echographically dyshomogeneous mass;

(3) Response to analogue treatment: all reported cases failed to respond and the mass continued to grow.

Two recent reports indicate that leiomyosarcomas can occur in women below the age of 40 years [55] and that degeneration can take place even in fibroids which originally responded to analogue treatment[65]. Figure 1 shows the appearance of a myoma which showed sudden growth, after 7 months of successful treatment with goserelin, and was, therefore, immediately operated. Figure 2 shows the appearance of one of the abdominal metastases which became evident 3 months after hysterectomy, causing a rapid exitus.

Association with hematological disorders

A rare but intriguing phenomenon, occasionally associated with the presence of leiomyomas, is erythrocytosis, a secondary isolated polycythemia usually seen in women in their fifties harboring a large myoma. Surgical removal of the tumor is followed by rapid disappearance of the condition[66,67]. Possible explanations for this association are the production of erythropoietin by the tumor[68], or the presence of extramedullary hematopoiesis within the context of the fibroid mass[69,70]. Erythropoietic activity has also been found in cutaneous leiomyomas[71]. Isolated reports have described additional associations between fibroids and the following hematological disorders: thrombocytopenia[72], chronic consumptive coagulopathy[73] and autoimmune thrombopenic purpura[74].

Treatment options

Since the first successful report of myomectomy by Atlee in 1845[75], surgery has represented the only viable option for treating uterine fibroids, although a variety of strange modalities have been utilized in the past[76]. Attempts to develop a medical therapy of leiomyomas began in 1946 when Goodman[77] reported that, in seven women, administration of progesterone produced a decrease in the size of the tumor or of the uterus in all cases treated, although Segaloff[78] failed to confirm this positive effect. The next step was the

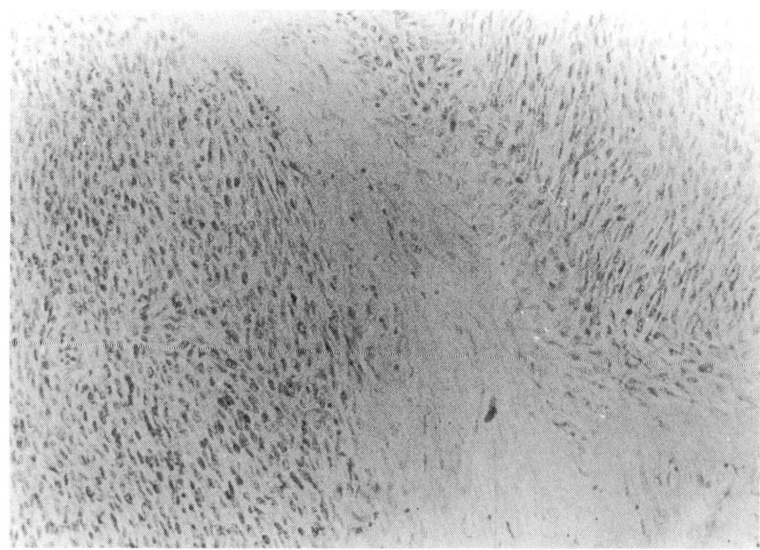

Figure 1 Histological appearance of a myoma which, after 7 months of successful treatment with goserelin, showed sudden growth and was, therefore, immediately operated

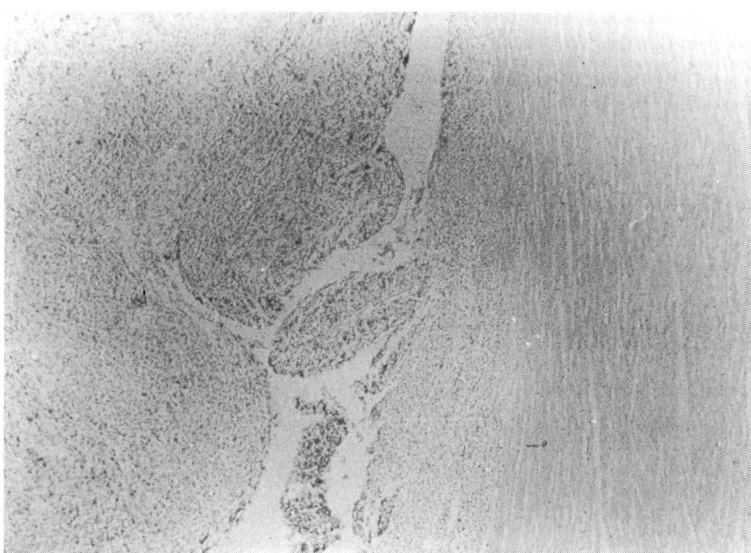

Figure 2 Same case as in Figure 1. Histological appearance of one of the abdominal metastases which became evident 3 months after hysterectomy

demonstration that the growth of leiomyomas can be blocked and red degeneration induced, using large doses of orally active, synthetic progestational steroids[47]. More recently, decrease in fibroid volume was also observed using two different antiprogestational steroids: gestrinone and mifepristone[79,80]. Treatment with analogues was only initiated in 1983, when, for the first time, a leiomyoma was shrunk and severe metrorrhagia stopped following pituitary desensitization[81]. This led to systematic research on the possibility of finding a medical treatment for uterine leiomyomas.

At least five comprehensive articles have recently reviewed treatment options for leiomyomas[21,51,58,76,82], discussing the major indications for GnRHa. During the Third International Symposium on GnRH Analogues in Cancer and Human Reproduction, three presentations dealt with this general topic [46,55,59].

It must be stressed that treatment for uterine fibroids is indicated only when – because of volume or location – tumors produce pain, menorrhagia and compression, or cause infertility. Whereas therapy must distinguish between young patients wishing to preserve or restore their fertility and older women who have completed their reproductive cycle, it is not uncommon in these days to receive requests for simple myomectomy from women above 40 who wish, if at all possible, that their uterus and ovaries be spared[82]. In this connection, a proper information campaign can decrease the incidence of hysterectomy in a community by 25%[83].

Rationally, use of GnRHa can be advocated in five different situations:

(1) As an adjunct before laparotomic hysterectomy;

(2) As an adjunct before laparotomic myomectomy;

(3) As an adjunct before laparoscopic myomectomy;

(4) As an adjunct to hysteroscopic myomectomy;

(5) As an alternative to surgery.

The role of GnRH analogues in laparotomic hysterectomy

Notwithstanding several attempts at medical treatment using progestogens[47,77,78], danazol[84–88], gestrinone[79,80] and gossypol[89], to this day hysterectomy remains the most widely utilized technique in women not wishing to have children, and the most frequently performed gynecological operation[90].

The substantial shrinkage of the vast majority of leiomyomas following therapy with GnRHa and the success of this therapy in completely blocking meno-metrorrhagias raised hope that surgery could be avoided altogether in many older women. Unfortunately, it has been amply documented that, once the effect of the agonist is reverted, the volume of both the tumor and the uterus rapidly return to their pretreatment size[91]. This is followed, in the majority of the patients, by recurrence of symptoms[92,93].

For this reason GnRHa treatment is now being proposed as adjunct therapy before hysterectomy[94]. There are only two real motives that justify the preoperative use of an analogue when hysterectomy for fibroids has been decided. The first is severe anemia: in a study of 16 women with a mean pretreatment hemoglobin concentration of 7.4 g/dl, levels rose to a mean of 13.2 g/dl after 3 months of treatment with goserelin[95]. In another study by our group, anemia was in nine cases severe enough to have caused hemoglobin concentrations to fall to 8 g/100 ml or below. The use of the GnRH analogue rapidly improved the situation, as shown in Figure 3. Hysterectomy was performed uneventfully in seven women: surgery became unnecessary in the remaining two patients[82]. Therefore, it can be stated that pretreatment with GnRH analogues is specifically indicated in subjects with severe anemia due to menorrhagia of long duration.

The question, however, still remains as to what constitutes an anemic condition 'severe enough' to warrant pretreatment. It has been suggested that any woman with a hemoglobin concentration lower than 12.0 g/dl or a red cell concentration of less than 3×10^6/ml should fall into this category. No specific data support these arbitrary cut-off points. Indeed, in the series of 171 patients with fibroids treated with GnRH analogues in our Institute in the last 6 years, 134 (78.4%) suffered from metromenorrhagia but only 54.5% had a hemoglobin concentration lower than 12.0 g/dl.

The second reason for advocating pretreatment is to reduce blood loss during surgery: in a randomized, multicenter double-blind, placebo-controlled trial involving 71 women conducted in Edinburgh, a significant reduction in blood loss at hysterectomy has been observed after 3 months of goserelin treatment. The results show a reduction in the mean blood loss in the treated group of 130 ml; blood losses exceeding 500 ml were measured in only two women in the pretreated group compared with seven among the controls. Goserelin pretreatment also caused a preoperative rise in hemoglobin concentration and relief of menstrual symptoms while waiting for surgery[96].

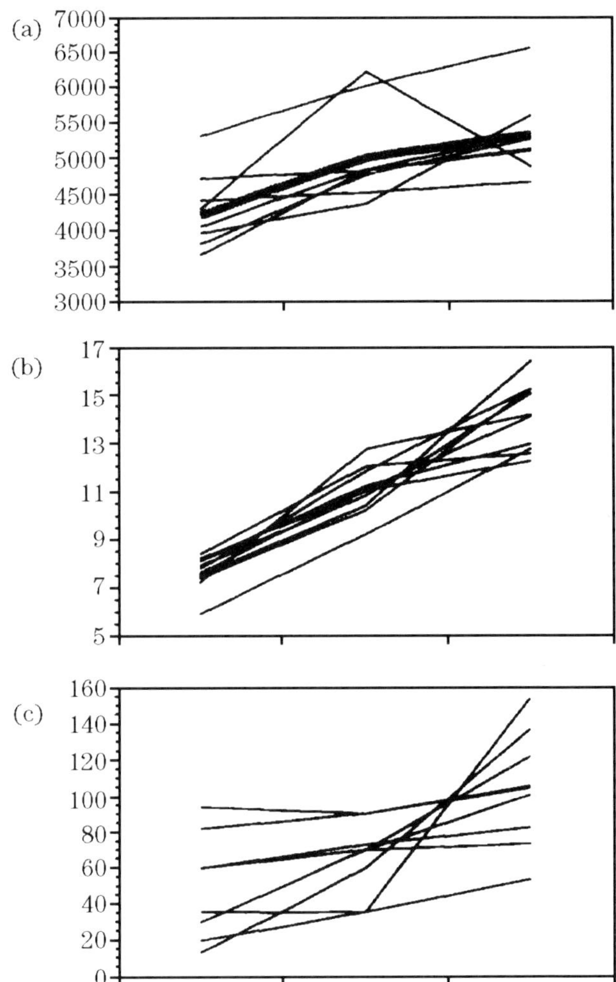

Figure 3 Hematological parameters in nine women with menometrorrhagia caused by uterine leiomyomata, before and after GnRH analogue treatment. (a) Red blood cells ($\times$ 1000/ml); (b) hemoglobin (g/dl); (c) blood iron

This clear advantage must be considered against the large cost of this therapy. Simply put, the question is: does a reduction of 100–150 ml in the blood loss during hysterectomy justify an extra expenditure of some $1000, and the postponement of the operation by 3–4 months?

In addition to these two well-defined conditions, there are other situations where pretreatment is deemed to be indicated on an individual basis, for example, when there are large broad ligament or cervical fibroids, or other factors that might make the operation technically difficult[97].

Pretreatment with GnRH analogues may also enable greater use of vaginal hysterectomy for patients with fibroids[98]. Stovall [42] compared 80 women with a pretreatment uterine size of 14–18 gestational weeks and 60 with uterine size greater than 18 weeks of gestation. He randomized patients in both groups to either immediate hysterectomy or 2 months' leuprolide therapy. Women with uteri 14/18 week size who received the agonist pre-operatively were significantly more likely to undergo vaginal hysterectomy (81% versus 13%; $p < 0.05$). In addition, these women had a shorter hospital stay, and a convalescence period. In contradistinction to this, in women with uteri larger than 18 weeks' gestational size, no difference could be observed between treated and non-treated cases. A shorter duration of surgery (49 versus 70 min) and a decrease in intraoperative blood loss (208 versus 309 ml) were also found by Golan and colleagues [48] when hysterectomy was preceded by decapeptyl administration.

The role of GnRH analogues in conservative surgical management

Much more complex is the evaluation of GnRH analogue pre- and/or post-treatment in the case of myomectomy, because we must distinguish between laparotomic, laparoscopic and hysteroscopic surgery.

Laparotomic myomectomy

Although a simple procedure, laparotomic myomectomy poses three types of problems: immediate bleeding requiring proper intraoperative hemostasis, the need to reconstruct uterine anatomy accurately, and the prevention of peritoneal adhesion and intrauterine sinechiae. In addition, in discussing GnRH adjunctive therapy, one must mention the need to eliminate every myomatous mass.

For each of these four points adjunctive treatment has both advantages and disadvantages:

(1) *Minimizing blood loss*   It is well proven today that the preoperative use of GnRH analogues has been a major advance in the minimization of

blood loss. Indeed, Doppler ultrasound has demonstrated significant changes occurring, under the influence of GnRH analogues, in uterine arterial blood flow velocity waveforms, with a parallel increase in the resistance index. In a now classic study[99], as the uterine arterial volume decreased from 656 to 386 ml, the uterine arterial resistance index increased from 0.52 to 0.92. In a controlled study, a strong correlation was found between total blood loss and size of the uterus in untreated subjects, but not in women pretreated with a GnRH analogue[100]. Analogue pretreatment is specifically indicated in subjects with severe anemia due to menorrhagia of long duration. As in the case of hysterectomy, the use of the analogue rapidly improves the situation, causing a substantial amelioration of hematological parameters.

Friedman and colleagues[100], in a double-blind, placebo-controlled study, were able to demonstrate that pretreatment with leuprolide acetate depot significantly reduced mean intraoperative blood loss, especially in patients with large uteri. In our experience, blood loss decreased from 255 ml (SD 53) in ten untreated controls, to 165 ml (SD 42) following GnRH analogue pretreatment in an additional ten patients[82].

On the other hand, Fedele and colleagues[101] could not find any significant difference in intraoperative blood loss between treated and untreated patients.

(2) *Ease at surgery and proper reconstruction of uterine anatomy*
Some surgeons have cast doubt on the wisdom of analogue pretreatment, in view of the fact that the fibroid 'capsule' becomes less evident, tumors do not 'shell out' cleanly, and the excision may be more difficult[100,102]. Others have defended the utility of pretreatment on general grounds, stating that the operation is easier[103], that there may be a better anatomical reconstruction, and that there is the possibility of utilizing Pfannenstiel transversal incision, even in the case of very large fibroids.

(3) *Prevention of peritoneal adhesions*   There is no reason to believe that analogue pre- or post-treatment can improve the situation. Therefore, one should continue to rely upon techniques such as microsurgery[104] and the use of CO_2, YAG or Argon lasers. Maheux[76] reports that, in laparotomic myomectomy, laser is unhelpful. On the contrary, others[105–108] believe that minimal blood loss, fewer adhesions and decreased anatomical disruption can improve long-term results, especially in infertile patients.

(4) *Ability to eliminate even the smaller myomas during surgery*
Some investigators and surgeons fear that small myomas may become invisible and, therefore, be left behind following surgery, exposing the patient to a greater risk of recurrence. Fedele and colleagues[101], in a small series of 24 women with symptomatic uterine myomas, found that pretreatment with buserelin significantly increased recurrence of leiomyomata (63% versus 13%) at 6 months.

Our group has attempted an overall assessment of the advantages and disadvantages of GnRH analogue pretreatment. To do so, 40 women were selected and randomly allocated either to immediate myomectomy, or to operation following 4 months of therapy with the GnRH analogue goserelin, administered as a depot formulation. From the patients submitted to immediate surgery, a total of 55 individual myomas were eventually excised, whereas the women pretreated with GnRH analogue therapy harbored 61 fibroids[82].

In general, surgery was judged to be easier in women pretreated with the analogue, although, using an arbitrary scoring system for several variables, only small differences were detected (total scores were 105.7 and 118.9 in pretreated and control patients, respectively). As a rule, the surgeon providing the score was not aware of whether the patient had been pretreated, although he was able to identify correctly the controls in 18 out of 20 cases. A sonographic evaluation 3 months after surgery did not show any major differences between the two groups, with a marginally better anatomical result achieved in pretreated subjects. Data are summarized in Figure 4.

In conclusion, data obtained so far have been unable to provide convincing facts on the superiority of conservative surgery, when carried out following pretreatment with GnRH analogues.

Steller and colleagues [49] followed-up myomectomies in a comparative, but not randomized, clinical trial to evaluate long-term results with or without analogue therapy. No statistically significant differences were observed between pretreated subjects and those directly operated. In both groups, pregnancy occurred in about one-third of the women wishing to conceive, and recurrence of myomas was observed in some 20% of the patients.

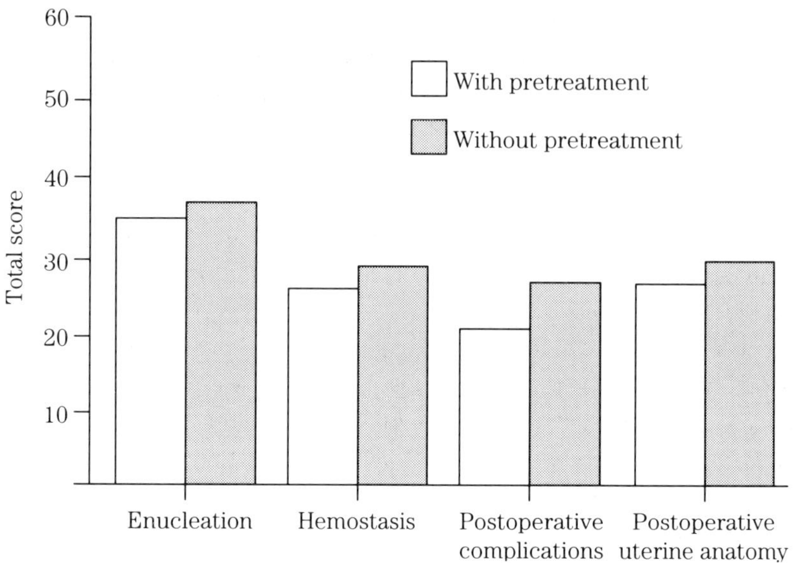

Figure 4 Arbitrary operative scoring utilized by the surgeon in myomectomies performed with or without pretreatment with a GnRH analogue (goserelin depot) in two groups of 20 women. The following subjective scoring system was utilized. Enucleation of individual tumors: 0.3, easy (manual); 0.6, medium (partially manual); 0.9, difficult (requiring instrumentation). The resulting scores were weighted to account for the difference in the total number of myomas (57 in treated and 61 in untreated patients). Hemostasis during operation: 1, good; 2, medium; 3, difficult. Postoperative complications: 1, none; 2, hyperthermia; 3, complications requiring prolongation of hospitalization. Postoperative anatomical reconstruction (as judged by ultrasound 3 months postsurgery): 1, normal volume and contour; 2, enlarged uterus with normal contour; 3, abnormal volume and altered contour

Laparoscopic myomectomy

This procedure is at present only utilized in selected centers and by a handful of laparoscopists. It is this procedure where GnRH analogue pretreatment can, theoretically, provide the most definite advantages. Indeed, the decreased risk of bleeding and the decreased size of the tumor represent very definite advantages if the myoma is pedunculated or clearly subserosal. If, on the other hand, the tumor is well endowed in the uterine wall, then cleavage will probably be more difficult and excision more problematic.

Recently, the use of a GnRH analogue following laparoscopic myomectomy has been advocated to decrease uterine size and improve long-term results[109].

Mettler and Semm [39], in a non-comparative study, performed laparoscopic myomectomies in 150 patients and confirmed that excision was easier and with a minimum of blood loss. They utilized the local application of a vasoconstrictive agent (POR-8), ligatures, sutures, the myoma enucleator and the serrated-edge macromorcellator. In another non-comparative study, Dubuisson and colleagues [141] removed, through operative laparoscopy, myomas in 95 women pretreated with a GnRH analogue. Following excision using monopolar coagulation, they removed the masses either by suprapubic incision or by colpotomy.

The introduction of video-endoscopy will probably allow more centers to carry out myomectomies and possibly amplify indications for endoscopic removal, which today are still limited. Indeed, leiomyomas having a diameter larger than 3 cm, located deep in the myometrium, especially if in the posterior side, cannot normally be removed through laparoscopy.

It is also possible that the utilization of laser techniques may provide further improvements[108].

Hysteroscopic myomectomy

Neuwirth and Amin[110] were the first in 1976 to excise submucous fibroids transcervically, under hysteroscopic control. Small or pedunculated tumors can be excised using standard procedures, whereas larger ones can be 'shaved' off using the resectoscope[21].

In the last few years, several groups have utilized pretreatment with a GnRH analogue in these patients[111–113]. It seems that the absence of bleeding can be an advantage; also, a decreased size could facilitate removal. On the other hand, several potential disadvantages can be envisaged: the shrinking of the uterus can make the procedure more difficult, non-pedunculated fibroids can retreat into the myometrium, and their excision could become impossible.

The combination of operative hysteroscopy and GnRH analogue pretreatment has been pioneered by Donnez[114]. Recently, he and his collaborators[115] treated 112 patients with submucosal fibroids, the greatest diameter of which was inside the cavity, performing myomectomy by hysteroscopy and Nd–YAG laser, and reported that the operation was relatively easy in all but two cases. The myometrium overlying the myoma was less vascular and the 'shrinkage' of the uterine cavity may have accounted for the relative ease of separating the myoma from the surrounding myometrium. In the two patients in whom the first operation was unsuccessful, a second hysteroscopy was performed 8 weeks later and the myoma successfully removed from the myometrium.

In patients with very large submucosal fibroids, of which the largest portion is not inside the uterine cavity but well inside the uterine wall, a two-step operative hysteroscopy has been proposed[115]. After 8 weeks of preoperative GnRH agonist therapy, a partial myomectomy is carried out by resecting the protruded portion of the myoma. Thereafter, the laser fiber is directed, as perpendicularly as possible, to the remaining (intramural) fibroid portion and introduced into the mass to a length of 5–10 mm. During the application of laser energy, the fiber is removed slowly so that the deeper areas are coagulated. Following completion of the procedure, therapy with the GnRH agonist is continued for another 8 weeks, and then a second-look hysteroscopy is performed. At this stage, usually, the shrinkage of the uterine cavity allows an easy dissection of the residual portion of myoma.

Several new studies have now been conducted: non-randomized controls were used by Perino and colleagues [40] who found that the duration of surgery, intraoperative bleeding and the amount of distension medium were reduced in patients pretreated with leuprolide. Donnez [58] has shown that the reduced vascularization induced by analogue treatment will also reduce the amount of distension medium absorbed and, therefore, the risk of fluid overflow. Corson [47] believes that GnRH analogue pretreatment may successfully decrease the size of submucous myomas large enough to almost fill the cavity, thereby enabling hysteroscopic surgery in cases where otherwise maneuvering a resectoscope might be impossible. Finally, Wallwiener and colleagues [43] prefer electroresection to the use of laser for large or non-pedunculated myomas.

GnRH analogues as an alternative to surgery

There is agreement among clinicians and researchers that analogue treatment should not normally be continued beyond 6 months. The problem, therefore, exists on how to maintain the good results obtained through GnRH analogue use, without keeping women in a condition of severe hypoestrogenism.

Essentially, two approaches have been taken: Friedman and colleagues[116] and Maheux[76] have treated women with an analogue until the size of the uterus and that of leiomyomas have properly diminished; then, while continuing the analogue, they added small quantities of an estrogen, followed by a progestin, as in hormonal replacement therapy. This regimen allows the disappearance of the negative side-effects associated with the analogue, without causing fibroid re-growth. More recently, the use of medroxyprogesterone acetate (MPA) without estrogen has been advocated. West and colleagues [56] tested the addition of MPA 15 mg/day after 3 months of goserelin administration. The progestogen greatly decreased the incidence of hypoestrogenic side-effects without causing any fibroid regrowth; unfortunately, patients experienced a consistent fall in bone mineral density. Opposite results have been reported by Carr and colleagues [54], who found that the addition of MPA at the dose of 20 mg/day caused re-growth of myomas but, at least partially, prevented bone mineral loss.

An interesting approach has been attempted by Broekmans and colleagues [53], who utilized complete, followed by partial, pituitary suppression, so decreasing the dose of triptorelin administered. Preliminary results show that the beneficial effects of the initial high-dose agonist treatment on uterine leiomyomas can be preserved by continuing low-dose supplementation.

The real criticism of this approach is its cost: 1 month of analogue therapy amounts to some $300; if treatment has to be continued for several years, surgery would certainly become more economical. This should be taken into account, although, in the overall picture, one should also consider the negative psychological consequences of hysterectomy[117].

Serra and colleagues [41] believe that, in woman candidates to surgery for symptomatic myomas, the simple use of leuprolide for 6 months may not only postpone surgery, but even eliminate, in some cases, the need for the operation, by converting a symptomatic into an asymptomatic condition.

Our group has treated 152 women, aged 40 or more, during 6 months with the GnRH analogue buserelin and goserelin-depot, trying a different approach: maintain the results of analogue therapy with the administration of medroxyprogesterone acetate after the agonist has been discontinued[86] through the administration to 62 women of MPA, either at doses decreasing from 200 to 25 mg, or at the fixed dosage of 200 mg.

Sequential GnRH analogue/MPA at decreasing doses

This has been tried in a total of 23 subjects, according to the following scheme: 200 mg the 1st month, 100 mg the 2nd, 50 mg the 3rd and 4th month, and 25 mg thereafter. As a first step, 36 women, having completed 6 months of buserelin therapy, were randomly assigned to two distinct groups: the first to be used as controls and the second to be given MPA[50].

Considering the effect on the uterus, buserelin produced a highly significant reduction ($p < 0.001$), followed, in the control group, by a highly significant re-growth after discontinuation of buserelin therapy ($p < 0.001$). In the group treated sequentially with MPA, buserelin also reduced the uterine volume in a highly significant manner ($p < 0.001$). At the end of MPA medication, significant re-growth of the uterus ($p < 0.01$) was observed, whereas a different picture emerged when analyzing the effects on fibroids. Under medication with buserelin, leiomyomas in the control group showed a highly significant decrease ($p < 0.025$); during the 6 months following discontinuation of treatment, there was, as expected, a highly significant increase ($p < 0.001$). In the group subsequently treated with MPA, buserelin also produced a highly significant reduction ($p < 0.01$); thereafter, during medication with MPA, re-growth was not significant ($p > 0.03$). Data for all 23 women treated with decreasing doses of MPA[118] are summarized in Figure 5.

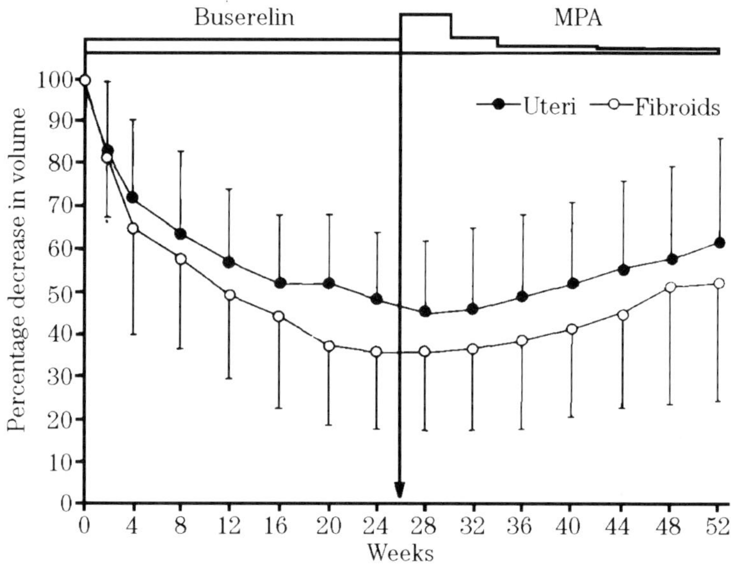

Figure 5 Mean percentage changes in the size of the uterus and of measurable leiomyomata following sequential buserelin–medroxyprogesterone acetate (MPA) treatment. Buserelin was administered to 23 women over 6 months. This was followed by 6 months of MPA at doses from 200 to 25 mg/day. For uteri, $p < 0.01$; for fibroids $p > 0.3$

In 11 women, treatment was continued for 1 year and in six and four, respectively, for 18 and 24 months. Briefly, whereas uteri progressively returned to their pretreatment volume, leiomyomas remained smaller. Overall, six of these patients (26.1%) have required hysterectomy so far. Surgical specimens from these six women were analyzed and areas of red degeneration were found in half of them.

Sequential GnRH analogue/MPA at fixed dosage

In order to improve results and shorten MPA treatment, a fixed dosage of 200 mg daily for a period of 6 months is being tried. To date, 39 patients have been included in this protocol but only eight completed the 6 months of MPA therapy. These women are being followed up without further medication. Interim results suggest that only some myomas do not regrow using this kind of treatment.

Several other sequential regimens have been tested in small groups of women. These include estriol at the dose of 4 mg per day, tamoxifen at the dose of 60 mg daily, and ethinylestradiol (20 µg) plus desogestrel (150 µg) for periods of 21 days followed by a 7-day interval. The results with all these regimens are so far inconsistent: uterine and fibroid re-growth have taken place.

Proposed classification of fibroids

Given the large amount of data collected by investigators in different parts of the world, a classification has been suggested for the description of the uterus and individual masses in cases of leiomyomas.

The classification should be based on a scoring system which could include the following variables:

(1) Localization;

(2) Number;

(3) Size;

(4) Thickness of the endometrium (phase to be determined);

(5) Symptomatology (bleeding, pain, urinary symptoms, etc.);

(6) Other associated lesions (endometriosis, adenomyosis, etc.);

(7) Association with infertility;

(8) Recurrency;

(9) General conditions of the patients (anemia);

(10) Blood flow through the uterus and myomas.

ENDOMETRIAL ABLATION

In cases of severe bleeding in women not desirous of pregnancy, endometrial ablation by laser vaporization represents an alternative to surgery, in subjects with normal or enlarged uteri[119].

The use of GnRH analogues before undertaking the hysteroscopic ablation has been recommended to reduce the hyperplastic endometrium, inevitably found in these patients, to an inactive one and therefore reduce intraoperative bleeding and fluid re-absorption.

Abramovich and colleagues [57] have carried out a preliminary comparative, randomized trial and found that the combination of GnRH analogue pretreatment and endometrial ablation, was, for the majority of the patients, a satisfactory alternative to hysterectomy.

In another preliminary trial, Corson [94] found that analogue treatment for just 1 month produces histologically better results than either progestins or danazol.

NEW CLINICAL INDICATIONS

During the meeting, a number of reports summarized preliminary experience of several new indications for GnRH analogue treatment in women.

Blumenfeld and colleagues [92] have successfully treated cyclic severe attacks of bronchial asthma, which required multiple hospitalization and even mechanical ventilation, in a 45-year-old woman using decapeptyl for 8 months. During treatment, the spirometric evaluation improved significantly, with an increase in the forced expiratory volume per second from 41.6 to 60.5% after 3 months. In another woman, they successfully employed the analogue in treating a number of neurological symptoms, appearing around menstruation and due to the presence of a thalamic hemangioma. After four injections of decapeptyl, the patient became asymptomatic and the beneficial effects persisted for several months.

Blumenfeld and colleagues [92] have also treated with GnRH analogue women of reproductive age with lymphoma, in the hope of reducing ovarian sensitivity to chemo- and/or radiotherapy. The first of these patients started menstruating after completing their different therapeutic regimens,

Analogues have also been employed by Calaf and colleagues [93] to treat menorrhagia in young women with bone marrow transplant; by Kinoshita and co-workers [95] as short-term treatment of clomiphene-resistant amenorrhea; by Barnan and colleagues [97] as an alternative to bromocriptine in women with macro- or micro/prolactinomas; and by Wiedeman and Stukensen [102] prior to cathcter dilatation in case of tubal nodular occlusion.

Finally Leonov and colleagues [101] have given decapeptyl to women with ovarian hyperstimulation syndrome. As expected, the analogue caused a worsening of the situation.

REFERENCES

1. Smith, C. J. (1952). Hysterectomy for benign pelvic conditions. *Am. J. Obstet. Gynecol.*, **64**, 1211–21
2. Rosai, J. (1989). *Ackerman's Surgical Pathology*, pp. 1083–7. (St. Louis: CV Mosby)
3. Torpin, R., Pund, E. and Peeples, W. J. (1942). The etiologic and pathologic factors in a series of 1,741 fibromyomas of the uterus. *Am. J. Obstet. Gynecol.*, **44**, 569–74
4. Rubenstein, A. H., Seftel, H. C., Miller, K., Berson, I. and Wright, A. D. (1969). Metabolic response to oral glucose in healthy South African white, Indian and African subjects. *Br. Med. J.*, **1**, 748–51
5. Miller, N. F. and Ludovici, P. P. (1955). On the origin and development of uterine fibroids. *Am. J. Obstet. Gynecol.*, **70**, 720–40
6. Ross, R. K., Pike, M. C., Vessey, M. P., Bull, D., Yeates, D. and Casagrande, J. T. (1986). Risk factors for uterine fibroids: reduced risk associated with oral contraceptives. *Br. Med. J.*, **293**, 359–62
7. John, A. H. and Martin, R. (1971). Growth of leiomyomata with estrogen–progestogen therapy. *J. Reprod. Med.*, **6**, 56–8
8. Lockyer, C. (1918). *Fibroids and Allied Tumours*, pp. 1–2. (London: MacMillan)
9. Townsend, D. E., Sparkes, R. S., Baluda, M. C. and McClelland, G. (1970). Unicellular histogenesis of uterine leiomyomas as determined by electrophoresis of glucose-6-phosphate dehydrogenase. *Am. J. Obstet. Gynecol.*, **107**, 1168–73

10. DeSnoo, K. (1934). The regeneration of the uterine mucosa in connection with myomata and endometriosis. *J. Obstet. Gynaecol. Br. Emp.*, **41**, 568–73

11. Meyer, R. (1930). In Henke and Lubarsch (eds.) *Handbuch der speciellen pathologischen Anatomie und Histologie.* (Berlin: Springer)

12. Stewart, M. J. (1935). Simple tumours of the uterus. In Teacher, G. H. (ed.) *Obstetrical and Gynaecological Pathology.* (London: Oxford University Press)

13. Zettergren, L. (1956). Histogenesis of uterina myomata. *Acta Obstet. Gynecol. Scand.*, **35**, 366–74

14. Heim, S., Nilvert, M., Vanni, R., Floderus, U., Mandahl, N., Liedgren, S., Lecca, U. and Nitelman, F. (1988). A specific translocation, t(12; 14) (q14-15; q23–24), characterizes a subgroup of uterine leiomyomas. *Cancer Genet. Cytogenet.*, **32**, 13–17

15. Gibas, Z., Griffin, G. A. and Emanuel, B. S. (1988). Clonal chromosome rearrangements in a uterine leiomyoma. *Cancer Genet. Cytogenet.*, **32**, 19–24

16. Turc-Carel, C., Dal Cin, P., Boghosian, L., Terk-Zakarian, J. and Sandberg, A. A. (1988). Consistent breakpoint in region 14 q22-24 in uterine leiomyoma. *Cancer Genet. Cytogenet.*, **32**, 25–31

17. Mugneret, F., Lizard-Nacol, S., Volk, C., Cuisenier, J., Colin, F. and Turc-Carel, C. (1988). Association of breakpoint 14q23 with uterine leiomyoma. *Cancer Genet. Cytogenet.*, **34**, 201–6

18. Vanni, R., Nieddu, M., Paoli, R. and Lecca, U. (1989). Uterine leiomyoma cytogenetics. I. Rearrangements of chromosome 12. *Cancer Genet. Cytogenet.*, **37**, 49–54

19. Boghosian, L., Dal Cin, P. and Sandberg, A. A. (1988). An interstitial deletion of chromosome 7 may characterize a subgroup of uterine leiomyoma. *Cancer Genet. Cytogenet.*, **34**, 207–8

20. Jani Sait, S. N., Dal Cin, P., Ovanessoff, S. and Sandberg, A. A. (1989). A uterine leiomyoma showing both t(12;14) and del(7) abnormalities. *Cancer Genet. Cytogenet.*, **37**, 157–61

21. Vollenhoven, B. J., Lawrence, A. S. and Healy, D. L. (1990). Uterine fibroids: a clinical review. *Br. J. Obstet. Gynaecol.*, **97**, 285–98

22. Wisot, A., Neimand, K. M. and Rosenthal, A. H. (1969). Symptomatic myoma in a 13-year-old girl. *Am. J. Obstet. Gynecol.*, **105**, 639–41

23. Milia, S., Lo Dico, G., Firinu, C., Mastinu, M. and Stoppelli, I. (1980). Su di un caso di leiomioma uterino in una giovane donna di 17 anni. *Min. Ginec.*, **32**, 909–11

24. Zaloudek, C. and Norris, H. J. (1987). Mesenchymal tumors of the uterus. In Kurman, R. G. (ed.) *Blaunstein's Pathology of the Female Genital Tract*, 3rd edn., pp. 373–408. (New York: Springer-Verlag)

25. Anderson, J. N., Peck, E. J. and Clark, J. H. (1975). Estrogen-induced uterine responses and growth: relationship to receptors-estrogen binding by uterine nuclei. *Endocrinology*, **96**, 160–7

26. Puukka, M. J., Kontula, K. K., Kauppila, A. J. J., Janne, O. A. and Vihko, R. K. (1976). Estrogen receptor in human myoma tissue. *Mol. Cell. Endocrinol.*, **6**, 35–44

27. Pollow, K., Geilfuss, J., Boquoi, E. and Pollow, B. (1978). Estrogen and progesterone binding proteins in normal human myometrium and leiomyoma tissue. *J. Clin. Chem. Clin. Biochem.*, **16**, 503–11

28. Tamaya, T., Motoyama, T., Ohono, Y., Ide, N., Tsurusaki, T. and Okada, H. (1979). Estradiol 17β, progesterone, and 5-alpha-dihydrotestosterone receptors of uterine myometrium and myoma in the human subject. *J. Steroid Biochem.*, **10**, 615–22

29. Buchi, K. and Keller, P. J. (1980). Estrogen receptors in normal and myomatous human uteri. *Gynecol. Obstet. Invest.*, **11**, 59–60

30. Wilson, E. A., Yang, F. and Rees, E. D. (1980). Estradiol and progesterone binding in uterine leiomyomata and in normal uterine tissue. *Obstet. Gynecol.*, **55**, 20–4

31. Soules, M. R. and McCarty, K. S. Jr. (1982). Leiomyomas: steroid receptor content. Variation within normal menstrual cycles. *Am. J. Obstet. Gynecol.*, **143**, 6–11

32. Sadan, O., van Iddekinge, B., Savage, N., Robinson, M. and Zakul, H. (1988). Ethnic variation in estrogen and progesterone receptor concentration in leiomyoma and normal myometrium. *Gynecol. Endocrinol.*, **2**, 275–82

33. Baird, D T., Bramley, T. A., Hawkins, T. A., Lumsden, M. A. and West, C. P. (1989). Effect of treatment with LHRH analogue Zoladex on binding of oestradiol, progesterone and epidermal growth factor to uterine fibromyomata. *Hormone Res.*, **32** (Suppl. 1), 154–6

34. Kornyei, J., Csermely, T., Szekely, J. A. and Vertes, M. (1986). Two types of nuclear E2 binding sites in human myometrium and leiomyoma during the menstrual cycle. *Exp. Clin. Endocrinol.*, **29**, 256–64

35. Otsuka, H., Shinohara, M., Kashimara, M., Yoshida, K. and Okamura, Y. (1989). A comparative study of the estrogen receptor ratio in myometrium and uterine leiomyomas. *Int. J. Gynecol. Obstet.*, **29**, 189–94

36. Spellacy, W. N., LeMaire, W. J., Buhl, W. C., Birk, S. A. and Bradley, B. A. (1972). Plasma growth hormone and estradiol levels in women with uterine myomas. *Obstet. Gynecol.*, **40**, 829–34

37. Maheux, R., Lemay-Turcot, L. and Lemay, A. (1986). Daily follicle-stimulating hormone, luteinizing hormone, estradiol, and progesterone in ten women harboring uterine leiomyomas. *Fertil. Steril.*, **46**, 205–8

38. Deligdish, L. and Loewenthal, M. (1970). Endometrial changes associated with myomata of the uterus. *J. Clin. Pathol.*, **23**, 676–80

39. Farrer-Brown, G., Beilby, J. O. W. and Tarbit, M. H. (1970). The vascular patterns in myomatous uteri. *J. Obstet. Gynaecol. Br. Commonw.*, **77**, 967–75

40. Yamamoto, T., Urabe, M., Naitoh, K., Kitawaki, J., Honjo, H. and Okada, H. (1990). Estrone sulfatase activity in human uterine leiomyoma. *Gynecol. Oncol.*, **37**, 315–18

41. Pollow, K., Sinnecker, G., Boquoi, E. and Pollow, B. (1978). *In vitro* conversion of estradiol-17-beta into estrone in normal human myometrium and leiomyoma. *J. Clin. Chem. Clin. Biochem.*, **16**, 493–52

42. Pasqualini, J. R., Cornier, E., Grenier, J., Vella, C., Schatz, B. and Netter, A. (1990). Effect of Decapeptyl, an agonistic analog of gonadotropin-releasing hormone on estrogens, estrogen sulfates, and progesterone receptors in leiomyoma and myometrium. *Fertil. Steril.*, **53**, 1012–17

43. Buchi, K. and Kekker, P. J. (1983). Cytoplasmic progestin receptors in myomal and myometrial tissues. *Acta Obstet. Gynecol. Scand.*, **62**, 487–92

44. Gorodeski, I. G., Geier, A., Beery, R., Bahary, C. M., Neri, A. and Lunenfeld, B. (1986). Characterization of the nuclear progesterone receptor in human uterine leiomyoma. *Eur. J. Gynecol. Reprod. Med.*, **23**, 91–9

45. Gorodeski, I. G., Bahary, C. M., Beery, R., Geier, A., Neri, A. and Lunenfeld, B. (1987). Decreased induced retention of the progesterone receptor in the nuclear extract in human uterine leiomyoma *in vivo*. *Gynecol. Obstet. Invest.*, **23**, 241–6

46. Navarro, D., Cabrera, J. J., Falcon, O., Jimenez, P., Ruiz, A., Chirino, R., Lopez, A., Rivero, J. F., Diaz-Chico, J. C. and Diaz-Chico, B. N. (1989). Monoclonal antibody characterization of progesterone receptors and the stress-responsive protein of 27 kDa (SRP27) in human uterine leiomyoma. *J. Steroid. Biochem.*, **34**, 491–8

47. Goldzieher, J. W., Maqueo, M., Ricaud, L., Aguilar, J. A. and Canales, E. (1966). Induction of degenerative changes in uterine myomas by high-dosage progestin therapy. *Am. J. Obstet. Gynecol.*, **96**, 1078–87

48. Faulkner, R. L. (1947). Red degeneration of uterine myomas. *Am. J. Obstet. Gynecol.*, **53**, 474–82

49. Friedman, A. J., Barbieri, R. L. and Doubilet, P. M. (1988). A randomized, double-blind trial of gonadotropin releasing-hormone agonist (leuprolide) with or without medroxyprogesterone acetate in the treatment of leiomyomata uteri. *Fertil. Steril.*, **49**, 404–9

50. Benagiano, G., Morini, A., Aleandri, V., Piccinno, F., Primiero, F. M., Abbondante, G. and Elkind-Hirsch, K. (1990). Sequential GnRH superagonist and medroxyprogesterone acetate treatment of uterine leiomyomata. *Int. J. Obstet. Gynecol.*, **33**, 333–43

51. Buttram, V. C. and Reiter, R. C. (1981). Uterine leiomyomata: etiology, symptomatology, and management. *Fertil. Steril.*, **36**, 433–45

52. Hofmann, G. E., Rao, V., Barrows, G. H., Schultz, G. S. and Sanfilippo, G. S. (1974). Binding sites for epidermal growth factors in human uteri tissues and leiomyomas. *J. Clin. Endocrinol. Metab.*, **58**, 880–3

53. Fayed, Y. M., Tsibris, J. C. M., Langenberg, P. W. and Robertson, A. L. Jr. (1989). Human uterine leiomyoma cells: binding and growth responses to epidermal growth factor, platelet-derived growth factor, and insulin. *Lab. Invest.*, **60**, 30–7

54. Lumsden, M. A., West, C. P., Bromley, J., Rumgay, L. and Baird, D. T. (1988). The binding of epidermal growth factor to the human uterus and leiomyoma in women rendered hypo-oestrogenic by continuous administration of an LH-RH-agonist. *Br. J. Obstet. Gynaecol.*, **95**, 1299–304

55. Koutsilieris, M., Michaud, J. and Nikolis, A. (1990). Preferential mitogenic activity for myoblast-like cells can be extracted from uterine leiomyoma tissues. *Am. J. Obstet. Gynecol.*, **163**, 1665–70

56. Wiznitzer, A., Marbach, M., Hazum, E., Insler, V., Sharoni, Y. and Levy, J. (1988). Gonadotrophin releasing hormone specific binding sites in uterine leiomyomata. *Biochem. Biophys. Res. Commun.*, **152**, 1326–31

57. Christopherson, W. M., Williamson, E. O. and Gray, L. A. (1972). Leiomyosarcoma of the uterus. *Cancer*, **29**, 1512–17

58. Buttram, V. C. Jr. (1986). Uterine leiomyomata – aetiology, symptomatology and management. In Rolland, R., Chadha, D. R. and Willemse, W. N. P. (eds.) *Gonadotropin Down-Regulation in Gynecological Practice. Progr. Clin. Biol. Res.*, **225**, 275–96

59. Leibsohn, S., d'Ablaing, G., Mishell, D. R. Jr. and Schlaerth, J. B. (1990). Leiomyosarcoma in a series of hysterectomies performed for presumed uterine leiomyomas. *Am. J. Obstet. Gynecol.*, **162**, 968–76

60. Baggish, M. S. (1974). Mesenchymal tumors of the uterus. *Clin. Obstet. Gynecol.*, **17**, 51–88

61. Hannigam, E. V. and Gomez, L. G. (1979). Uterine leiomyosarcoma: a review of prognostic clinical and pathologic features. *Am. J. Obstet. Gynecol.*, **134**, 557–64

62. Novak, E. R. and Woodruf, V. D. (1974). Myoma and other benign tumors of the uterus. In *Gynecologic and Obstetric Pathology*, 8th edn., p. 260. (Philadelphia: WB Saunders)

63. Loong, E. P. and Wong, F. W. (1990). Uterine leiomyosarcoma diagnosed during treatment with agonist of luteinizing hormone-releasing hormone for presumed uterine fibroid. *Fertil. Steril.*, **54**, 530–1

64. Meyer, W. R., Mayer, A R., Diamond, M. P., Carcangiu, M. L. and Schwartz, P. E. (1990). Unsuspected leiomyosarcoma: treatment with a gonadotropin-releasing hormone analogue. *Obstet. Gynecol.*, **75**, 529–32

65. Benagiano, G. and Morini, A. Unpublished data

66. Thomson, A. P. and Marson, F. G. W. (1953). Polycythaemia with fibroids. *Lancet*, **2**, 759–60

67. Jensen, K. R. (1990). Dyb tromboflebit ved polycytemi og fibromyoma uteri. *Ugeskr. Laeger*, **152**, 2316–18

68. Desablens, B., Steenkiste, G., Boffa, G. A. and Messerschmitt, J. (1980). Polycythemia and uterine fibroma. A case with *in vitro* demonstration of an erythropoietic activity in the tumor. *Sem. Hop. Paris*, **56**, 1138–44

69. Fadel de Tarsitano, M. I., Bianchi de Di Risio, C., Fernandez, J., Cagnacci, H. H. and Brieux de Salum, S. (1983). Deteccion de actividad eritropoyetica en celulas de un fibromioma. *Sangre*, **28**, 682–6

70. Schmid, C., Beham, A. and Kratochvil, P. (1990). Haematopoiesis in a degenerating uterine leiomyoma. *Arch. Gynecol. Obstet.*, **248**, 81–6

71. Venencie, P. Y., Puissant, A., Boffa, G. A., Sohier, J. and Duperrat, B. (1982). Multiple cutaneous leiomyomata and erythrocytosis with demonstration of erythropoietic activity in the cutaneous leiomyomata. *Br. J. Dermatol.*, **107**, 483–6

72. Dine, G., Dupoirieux, J., Hopfener, C. and Duhamel, G. (1984). Thrombopenie associée à un léiomyome utérin. Guérison aprés hystérectomie. *Press. Med.* (letter), **13**, 1459

73. Harris, M. G., Bannatyne, P., Russel, P., Atkinson, K., Rickard, K. A. and Kronenberg, H. (1982). Chronic consumptive coagulopathy with a uterine leiomyoma. *Aust. N.Z. J. Obstet. Gynaecol.*, **22**, 54–8

74. Duhamel, G., Dupoirieux, J., Hopfner, C., Dine, G. and Reznikoff, M. (1984). Association d'un purpura thrombopénique auto-immun et d'un léiomyome. Guérison après exerèse de la tumeur. *Press. Med.*, **13**, 2005–7

75. Atlee, W. L. (1845). Case of a successful extirpation of a fibrois tumor of the peritoneal surface of the uterus by the large peritoneal section. *Am. J. Med. Sci.*, **9**, 309–35

76. Maheux, R. (1990). Treatment of uterine leiomyomata: past, present and future. In Genazzani, A. R., Petraglia, F. and Volpe, A. (eds.) *Progress in Gynecology and Obstetrics*, pp. 173–90. (Carnforth, UK: Parthenon Publishing)

77. Goodman, A. L. (1946). Progesterone therapy in uterine fibromyoma. *J. Clin. Endocrinol.*, **6**, 402–8

78. Segaloff, A., Weed, J. C., Sternberg, W H. and Parson, D. (1949). The progesterone therapy of human uterine leiomyomas. *J. Clin. Endocrinol.*, **9**, 1273–91

79. Coutinho, E. M. (1981). Conservative treatment of uterine leiomyoma with the antiestrogen, antiprogesterone R-2323. *Int. J. Obstet. Gynecol.*, **19**, 557–60

80. Coutinho, E. M., Azadian-Boulanger, J. and Goncalves, M. T. (1986). Regression of uterine leiomyomas after treatment with gestrinone, an antiestrogen, anti-progesterone. *Am. J. Obstet. Gynecol.*, **155**, 761–7

81. Filicori, M., Hall, D. A., Loughlin, J. S., Rivier, J., Vale, W. and Crowley, W. F. Jr. (1983). A conservative approach to the management of uterine leiomyoma: pituitary desensitization by a luteinizing hormone-releasing hormone analogue. *Am. J. Obstet. Gynecol.*, **147**, 726–7

82. Benagiano, G., Morini, A. and Primiero, F. M. (1992). Fibroids: overview of current and future treatment options. *Br. J. Obstet. Gynaecol.*, **99** (Suppl. 7), 18–22

83. Domenighetti, G., Luraschi, P., Gutzwiller, F., Pedrinis, E., Casabianca, A., Spinelli, A. and Repatto, F. (1988). Effect of information campaign by the mass media on hysterectomy rates. *Lancet*, **2**, 1470–3

84. Yuen, B. H. (1981). Danazol and uterine leiomyomas. *J. Can. Med. Assoc.*, **124**, 963–4

85. de Cherney, A., Maheux, R. and Polan, M. L. (1983). A medical treatment for myomata uteri. *Fertil. Steril.*, **39**, 429–30

86. Benagiano, G., Morini, A., Abbondante, G., Isidori, C. and La Torre, P. C. (1987). Terapia del fibroleiomioma uterino. Risultati preliminari di une studio comparativo con danazolo, buserelin e medrossiprogesterone acetato. In Genazzani, A. R., Volpe, A. and Facchinetti, F. (eds.) *Ostetricia e ginecologia '87*, Vol. 2, pp. 9–19. (Roma: CIC Edizioni Internazionali)

87. Primiero, F. M., Morini, A., Abbondante, G., Caruso, G., Piccinno, F. and Benagiano, G. (1987). Terapia medica sequenziale del fibromioma uterino con danazolo e progestinici. In Fioretti, P. and Melis, G. B. (eds.) *Aggiornamenti in Scienze Ginecologioche ed Ostetriche*, pp. 879–87. (Roma: CIC Edizioni Internazionale)

88. Montemagno, U. and Nappi, C. (1987). Uso preoperatorio del danazolo nella terapia dei miomi uterini. In Fioretti, P. and Melis, G. B. (eds.) *Aggiornamenti in Scienze Ginecologiche ed Ostetriche*, pp. 205–10. (Roma: CIC Edizioni Internazionale)

89. Mei-ling, H. (1980). Gossipol treatment for menopausal functional bleeding, myoma of uterus and endometriosis: preliminary report. *Acta Acad. Med. Sin.*, **2**, 170–3

90. National Center for Health Statistics (1982). Utilization of shortstay hospitals. Annual summary for the United States 1980. Vital and Health Statistics Series 13, 64

91. Benagiano, G. (1989). Uterine fibroids: literature review and summary of posters. *Horm. Res.*, **32** (Suppl. 1), 120–4

92. Letteri, G. S., Shawker, T. H., Coddington, C. C., Loriaux, D. L., Winkel, C. A. and Collins, R. L. (1989). Efficacy of gonadotropin releasing hormone agonist

in the treatment of uterine leiomyomata: long-term follow-up. *Fertil. Steril.*, **51**, 951–6

93. Matta, W. H. M., Shaw, R. W. and Nye, M. (1989). Long-term follow-up of patients with uterine fibroids after treatment with the LHRH agonist buserelin. *Br. J. Obstet. Gynaecol.*, **96**, 200–6

94. Lumsden, M A., West, C. P. and Baird, D. T. (1987). Goserelin therapy before surgery for uterine fibroids. *Lancet*, **1**, 36–7

95. Candiani, G. B., Vercellini, P., Fedele, .P., Arcaini, L., Bianchi, S. and Candiani, M. (1990). Use of goserelin depot, a gonadotropin releasing hormone agonist, for the treatment of menorrhagia and severe anemia in women with leiomyomata uteri. *Acta Obstet. Gynecol. Scand.*, **69**, 413–15

96. Lumsden, M. A., Thomas, E., Coutts, J. R. T., West, C. P. and Baird, D. T. (1990). Goserelin pretreatment facilitates abdominal hysterectomy for the removal of uterine leiomyomata (fibroids). *Gynecol. Endocrinol.*, **4** (Suppl. 2), 41–4

97. West, C. P., Lumsden, M. A. and Baird, D. T. (1992). Goserelin (Zoladex) in the treatment of fibroids. *Br. J. Obstet. Gynaecol.*, **99** (Suppl. 7), 27–30

98. Stovall, T. G., Ling, F. W., Henry, L. C. and Woodruff, M. R. (1991). A randomized trial evaluating leuprolide acetate before hysterectomy as treatment for leiomyomas. *Am. J. Obstet. Gynecol.*, **164**, 1420–5

99. Matta, W. H. M., Stabile, I., Shaw, R. W. and Campbell, S. (1988). Doppler assessment of uterine blood flow changes in patients with fibroids receiving the gonadotropin releasing hormone agonist buserelin. *Fertil. Steril.*, **49**, 1083–5

100. Friedman, A. J., Rein, M. S., Harrison-Atlas, D., Garfield, J. M. and Doubilet, P. M. (1989). A randomized, placebo-controlled, double-blind study evaluating leuprolide acetate depot treatment before myomectomy. *Fertil. Steril.*, **52**, 728–33

101. Fedele, L., Vercellini, P., Bianchi, S., Brioschi, D. and Dorta, M. (1990). Treatment with GnRH agonists before myomectomy and the risk of short-term myoma recurrence. *Br. J. Obstet. Gynaecol.*, **97**, 393–6

102. Stovall, T. G. (1989). Rationale for the short-term use of luteinising hormone-releasing hormone analogues in the treatment of uterine myomata. *Horm. Res.*, **32** (Suppl. 1), 134–6

103. Editorial (1986). Uterine fibroids: medical treatment or surgery? *Lancet*, **2**, 1197

104. Corson, S. L. and Smith, D. C. (1980). Principles and instrumentation of microsurgery. *Clin. Obstet. Gynecol.*, **23**, 1201–14

105. McLaughlin, D. S. (1985). Metroplasty and myomectomy with the CO_2 laser for maximizing the preservation of normal tissue and minimizing blood loss. *J. Reprod. Med.*, **30**, 1–9

106. Reyniak, J. W, and Corenthal, L. (1987). Microsurgical laser technique for abdominal myomectomy. *Microsurgery*, **8**, 92–8

107. Starks, G. C. (1988). CO_2 laser myomectomy in an infertile population. *J. Reprod. Med.*, **33**, 184–6

108. March, C. M. (1989). Update: laser surgery. *Endocr. Fertil. Forum*, **9**, 1–5

109. Huber, J. C. (1990). Combined endoscopical and endocrinological treatment of uterine fibroids. In Vickery, B. H. and Lunenfeld, B. (eds.) *GnRH Analogues and Human Reproduction*, Vol. III, *Benign and Malignant Tumors*, pp. 63–5. (London: Kluwer Academic Publishers)

110. Neuwirth, R. S. and Amin, H. K. (1976). Excision of submucus fibroids with hysteroscopic control. *Am. J. Obstet. Gynecol.*, **126**, 95–9

111. Blanc, B., Boubli, L., Barry, I. and Bertrand, Y. (1989). Chirurgie des fibromes après traitement par analogue de la GnRH. Presented at the *II World Congress of Gynecology Endoscopy*, Clermont-Ferrand

112. Hourcabie, J. and Amouroux, M. (1989). Résection hysteroscopique des fibromes uterins après préparation par analogue de la GnRH. Presented at the *II World Congress of Gynecology Endoscopy*, Clermont-Ferrand

113. Lawrence, A. S., Healy, D. L., Hill, D. and Paterson, P. J. (1991). Management of a submucous uterine fibroid with buserelin, gemeprost and hysteroscopic resection. *Med. J. Aust.*, **154**, 280–2

114. Donnez, J., Sandow, J., Schurs, B., Clerckx, F. and Gillerot, S. (1989). Treatment of uterine fibroids with implants of gonadotropin releasing hormone agonist: assessment by hysterography. *Fertil. Steril.*, **51**, 947–50

115. Donnez, J., Nisolle, M., Grandjean, P., Gillerot, S. and Clerckx, F. (1992). The place of GnRH agonists in the treatment of endometriosis and fibroids by advanced endoscopic techniques. *Br. J. Obstet. Gynaecol.*, **99** (Suppl. 7), 31–3

116. Friedman, A. J. (1989). Treatment of leiomyomata uteri with short-term leuprolide followed by leuprolide plus estrogen-hormone replacement therapy for 2 years: a pilot study. *Fertil. Steril.*, **51**, 526–8

117. Richards, D. H. (1973). Depression after hysterectomy. *Lancet*, **2**, 430–3

118. Benagiano, G., Morini, A., Aleandri, V., Piccinno, F., Angelini, R. and Goldzieher, J. W. (1990). Sequential buserelin-medroxyprogesterone acetate treatment of leiomyomata uteri. In Brosens, I., Jacobs, H. S. and Runnebaum, B. (eds.) *LHRH Analogues in Gynaecology*, pp. 111–25. (Carnforth, UK: Parthenon Publishing)

119. Lomano, J. (1991). Endometrial ablation for the treatment of menorrhagia: a comparison of patients with normal, enlarged and fibroid uteri. *Lasers Surg. Med.*, **11**, 8–12

BIBLIOGRAPHY

Abstracts of relevant papers presented at the 3rd International Symposium on GnRH Analogues in Cancer and Human Reproduction

38. Immunohistochemical receptor status of the uterus and its fibroids. U. Cirkel, H. Ochs, A. Rochl, H. P. G. Schneider, Germany

39. Laparoscopic approach of fibroid excision after treatment with Gn-RH analogues. L. Mettler, K. Semm, Germany

40. Role of leuprolide acetate depot in hysteroscopic surgery: a controlled trial. A. Perino, N. Chianchiano, M. Petronio, E. Cittadini, Italy

41. Clinical follow up in patients with symptomatic leiomyomata uteri treated with leuprolide acetate depot. G. Serra, V. Panetta, D. Zampolla, S. Polverari, G. C. Giraldi, R. Fanfani, A. Biamonti, U. Epifani, Italy

42. GnRH agonist use prior to hysterectomy. T. G. Stovall, USA

43. Hysteroscopic approach of fibroids after pretreatment with GnRH agonists (GnRH-A). D. Wallwiener, S. Rimbach, D. Pollman, C. Sohn, T. Rabe, G. Bastert, Germany

45. The scientific rationale of management of uterine fibroids with GnRH analogues. G. Benagiano, Italy

46. Gonadotropin-releasing hormone analogs (agonists and antagonists) in the treatment of uterine leiomyomas: advantages and disadvantages. J. Cohen, France

47. Gonadotropin releasing hormone analogs prior to hysteroscopic myomectomy. S. L. Corson, USA

48. Preoperative GnRH-analog treatment in surgery for uterine myomas. A. Golan, D. Bukovsky, M. Schneider, M. Pansky, E. Caspi, Israel

49. Follow up investigations after myomectomy. J. Steller, K. Husch, E. Daume, Germany

50. Cytogenetic investigation of leiomyomas treated with the GnRH-analogue goserelin. U. Deichert, J. Bullerdick, Y. Hennig, M. van de Sandt, J. Nicolai, S. Helms, Germany

51. The effect of decapeptyl on the growth of leiomyomata. E. Johannisson, I. Brosens, P. Dalcin, Switzerland and Belgium

53. GnRH agonists treatment of uterine leiomyoma: complete followed by partial pituitary suppression. F. J. Broekmans, P. G. A. Hompes, J. Schoemaker, Netherlands

54. Effect of hormonal add-back therapy utilizing medroxyprogesterone acetate plus GnRH agonists on calcium balance and uterine leiomyomata. B. R. Carr, P. B. Marshburn, P. T. Weatherall, N. A. Breslau, M. P. Steinkampf, USA

55. Unsuspected leiomyosarcoma (intermediate grade) with metastasis in a patient on gonadotropin releasing hormone analogue for treatment of myomata. G. P. Gidwani, J. M. Goldberg, A. W. Kennedy, USA

56. Potential role of medroxyprogesterone acetate as an adjunct to zoladex in the medical management of uterine fibroids. C. West, L. Caird, J. Creiger, M. A. Lumsden, D. Baird, UK

57. Hysteroscopic treatment of dysfunctional uterine bleeding. D. R. Abramovich, S. Pinion, D. Parkin, H. Kitchener, G. Flett, P. Smith, UK

58. Large submucosal myoma: GnRH agonist and hysteroscopic myomectomy. J. Donnez, Belgium

59. The use of GnRH analogues in endometriosis and fibroids: adjunctive or alternative approach to surgery? R. Maheux, Canada

92. New clinical indications for GnRH analogues: Menstrual asthma, thalamic hemangioma, breast carcinoma, and lymphomas in young women. Z. Blumenfeld, L. Bentur, A. Rubin, J. Aaron, N. Haim, J. M. Brandes, Israel

93. GnRH analogues in the management of menorrhagia in bone marrow transplantation. J. Calaf, E. Capdevila, A. Altes, S. Brunet, C. Sola, Spain

94. Gonadotropin releasing hormone analogs prior to endometrial ablation. S. L. Corson, USA

95. Short term administration of GnRH agonist for treatment of hypogonadotrophic secondary amenorrhea. K. Kinoshita, O. Ishihara, Y. Iino, M. Saitoh, H. Seki, Japan

97. The effect of treatment with a GnRH analog and bromocriptine in patients with hyperprolactinemia. R. Barnan, A. Golan, N. Eckstein, S. Avidan, R. Limor, I. Vagman, D. Aylon, Israel

101. Peculiarities of OHSS course under decapeptyl daily injection and depo-forms application in ivf/et program. B. Leonov, V. Kulakov, K. Yavorovskaya, V. Smolnikova, E. Kalinina, R. Schedrina, N. Fanchenko, Russia

102. Proximal tubal occlusion-microsurgical repair or catheter dilatation? R. Wiedmann, J. Stuckensen, Germany

141. Gonadotropin-releasing hormone agonist and laparoscopic myomectomy. J. B. Dubuisson, C. Chapron, F. Lecuru, H. Foulout, F. X. Aubriot, J. Bouquet de Joliniere, France

6

GnRH analogues in precocious puberty and management of small-growing children

R. Kauli

The gonadotropin releasing hormone analogues (GnRHa) seem to have satisfactorily solved one of the most difficult therapeutic problems in pediatrics – the treatment of central precocious puberty. In this condition, a pubertal pattern of GnRH secretion starts significantly earlier than in the physiological age range, followed by an early increase of gonadotropin and gonadal steroid secretion and pubertal development at a very young age. It can be caused by various etiological factors although most frequently, particularly in girls, it is defined as idiopathic because no underlying organic disease can be found, even with the most advanced diagnostic techniques available at present.

The precocious sexual maturation is associated with an early increase of growth velocity and bone maturation rate, the latter being frequently inadequately accelerated. The affected children are tall as compared to their peers but their final height can be significantly compromised because of early closure of the bone epiphyses (Figure 1).

The objectives of treatment of central precocious puberty are twofold:

(1) To arrest further development of the pubertal signs which frequently cause significant emotional and psychosocial problems.

(2) To decrease growth velocity and bone maturation back to the prepubertal rate, and make possible the achievement of adult height in accordance with the genetic growth potential of the patient.

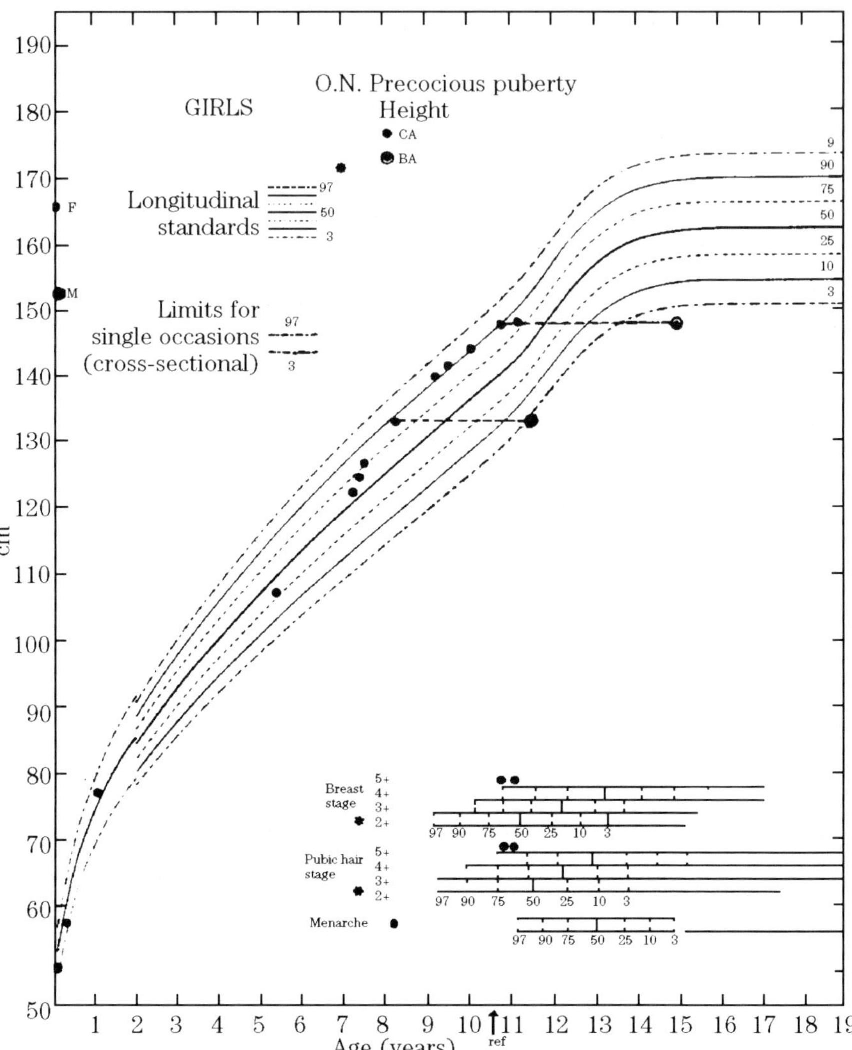

Figure 1 Growth chart of girl who developed idiopathic central precocious puberty at age 6 years and 6 months and was not treated, according to the family's decision. Menarche appeared at 9 years and she reached final height at age 10 years 10 months, below the mid-parental height

Before GnRHa were available, patients with central precocious puberty were treated with various synthetic progestational agents[1-10], which suppressed gonadotropin secretion but mostly uncompletely and in an unsustained manner. After the observation that synthetic superactive GnRH agonists[11] at first induce a transitory stimulation later followed by a sustained paradoxical inhibition of gonadotropin secretion[12], these compounds were introduced in clinical practice for the treatment of central precocious puberty[13–15]. Over a decade has passed and considerable experience has been achieved by now which has been published in the pediatric and endocrinological literature and discussed at international scientific meetings. The International Symposia on GnRH Analogues, which have taken place here in Geneva, have reflected and summarized periodically the accumulated knowledge and experience, as well as the unclarified issues and controversies.

Many studies have been published on the pharmacodynamics, on the effect on the clinical signs of puberty, on growth and bone maturation rate and on the changes in the hormonal status of children treated with the available preparations of GnRHa[16–37]. With time, long-term follow-up studies during and after therapy have been reported, with results on the subsequent resumption and completion of puberty, on gonadal function and subsequent growth, up to final height[38–53]. While the reversibility of gonadotropin suppression has been established and universally accepted, the benefit on achieved final height is still a controversial issue.

During the first few years after the introduction of the GnRHa therapy for central precocious puberty, the sustained, and yet reversible suppression of gonadotropin secretion and gonadarche, evident clinically and documented by laboratory examinations, was the main subject of research[16–37]. The experience achieved during those first years was presented and discussed at the 1st Symposium on GnRH Analogues in February 1988[32–36]. It was well established, at that time, that by daily administration of GnRHa, after a transitory stimulatory phase, gonadotropin secretion is suppressed by down-regulation of the GnRH receptor cells in the pituitary gland. This is followed by a sustained decrease of gonadal sex steroid secretion, down to prepubertal levels, and arrest of the gonadotropin-dependent pubertal signs (gonadarche), while adrenarche is unaffected[19,30,33,34]. The gonadotropin suppression is documented by suppressed values of basal as well as of GnRH-stimulated levels. We have found occasional increases of gonadotropin levels in treated patients but without any clinical evidence of escape from the state of pubertal suppression[33]. It can be assumed that these are biologically inactive but radioimmunoassay-detectable α-subunits of gonadotropins, which have been demonstrated[31,37]. The gonadotropin suppression caused by the GnRHa therapy was found to be fully reversible and, after its discontinuation, restoration of pubertal development was observed[24,35,38].

With the arrest of gonadarche in patients with central precocious puberty treated with GnRHa, marked decreases of growth velocity and of bone maturation rate are observed. These were found to be associated with a decrease of spontaneous growth hormone secretion back to the prepubertal rate[34], even if the growth hormone response to stimulatory tests remained unchanged[33]. A subsequent improvement of final height prognosis was reported, at that time based mainly on changes in the predicted final height of patients after longer periods of therapy[16,22,25,32].

At the 2nd Symposium on GnRH Analogues in November 1990, most of the presented studies reported more information on long-term follow-up with the therapy and on growth and pubertal development after it[40–50]. The reversibility of gonadotropin suppression was reconfirmed and encouraging data on post-therapy reactivation of gonadarche and on gonadal function were presented. More positive data were reported on the improvement of final height prognosis in central precocious puberty patients treated with GnRHa, as compared to historic untreated controls[40]. Most of the studies were based on predicted final height after therapy[40–42,45–47], but there were already some data on achieved final height[43]. The benefit on post-treatment predicted final height was found to correlate with the severity of central precocious puberty at the start of therapy[45]. The achieved final height was found to reach mid-parental height, i.e. the target height (Figure 2), if therapy was not started at a too advanced bone age[43].

Important experience was reported with rare forms of gonadotropin-independent and thus, GnRHa-resistant precocious puberty such as McCune–Albright syndrome in girls[54] and testotoxicosis in boys[55]. As expected, the GnRHa fails to suppress pubertal development in these syndromes, but it is of interest that it can help to elucidate their pathogenesis by confirming that gonadal hyperfunction in these patients is not of central origin, and other means of therapy have to be used.

Moreover, at the 2nd Symposium, preliminary research data on additional aspects of GnRHa were reported, such as their use as diagnostic agents in delayed puberty[56], and as complementary therapeutic agents in conventional[57] and in non-conventional growth hormone therapy[58].

During this 3rd symposium at the workshop on GnRHa in central precocious puberty, more studies on these additional aspects of GnRHa were reported, and, as expected additional information on long-term follow-up

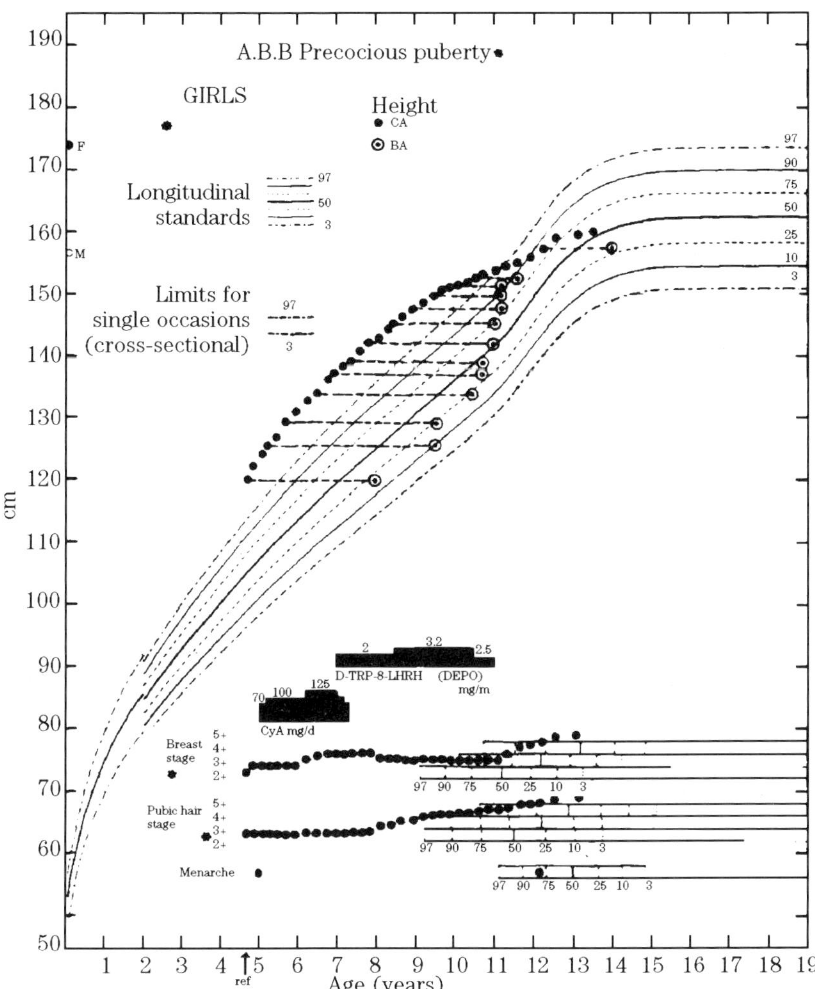

Figure 2 Growth chart of girl who developed idiopathic central precocious puberty at age 4 years 9 months with menarche at age 5 years. She was treated since the age of 5 years with cyproterone acetate; adrenarche was arrested but gonadarche became gradually resistant to this therapy, even with increasing dosage. Treatment was switched to GnRHa (intramuscular Decapeptyl®, i.e. D-Trp-6-LHRH-depo) at age 7 years. Subsequent gonadarche was arrested, growth velocity decreased to the prepubertal rate and bone maturation was almost arrested. Adrenarche reappeared at age 8 years but progressed at a rate appropriate for age. Therapy was discontinued at age 11 years 2 months and, thereafter, she completed her puberty and growth and her final height reached mid-parental height. Menarche reappeared at age 12 years 2 months

after therapy, such as final height and gonadal function after therapy, was presented and discussed.

LONG-TERM RESULTS IN CENTRAL PRECOCIOUS PUBERTY PATIENTS TREATED WITH GnRHa

Two studies were presented. In the first, Baens and Lee [125] reported on a study of the long-term results of GnRHa therapy in 25 children with central precocious puberty who had reached their final height. They found a resumption of pubertal activity of the hypothalamo–pituitary–gonadal axis and normal gonadal function in their patients after therapy. An important contribution from their study is the finding of normal bone density in the patients after therapy. However, the achieved final height of the patients, as compared to pre- and post-treatment predictions was not significantly affected.

The second study [129] reported a definite beneficial effect of therapy with GnRHa on the final height of girls with central precocious puberty. The benefit of therapy was evaluated by taking into consideration the genetic growth potential of the patients. It was found that 32 girls with precocious puberty treated with GnRHa as well as 28 girls with precocious puberty treated with cyproterone acetate achieved a final height within their genetic growth potential and significantly above the pretreatment prediction. A control group of 25 untreated girls with precocious puberty achieved a mean final height below mid-parental height and the distribution analysis revealed that half of them (12/25) ended up with a final height well below their expected genetic range and below the standard deviation score of both parents, because of a disproportionally accelerated bone maturation rate.

It is of note that no difference in final height achievements was found between therapy with cyproterone acetate and GnRHa. However, GnRHa therapy has the advantages of better compliance with the depot preparations and, according to our experience, no significant side-effects and no failures so far.

During the discussion of the presented results on final height, in treated and untreated girls with central precocious puberty, the difficult question about indication for and timing of therapy was raised. This question has been put forward in the past, and also at the 1st Symposium[59,60], arising from patients whose central precocious puberty is spontaneously arrested, unsustained or progresses very slowly, without progressive advancement of bone maturation. Such patients achieve a final height equal or close to their target height without any therapy. However, considering the possibility of a marked compromise of final height should the precocious pubertal process be accelerated, we feel that treatment should be decided upon after a limited period of follow-up, to avoid further advancement of bone age.

Of particular interest was the report by Gshwend and Lee [126] on six female infants (less than 2 years old) with central precocious puberty who were treated with GnRHa. The instigators reported the high incidence of tumors in the central nervous system (half of the patients) and the different diagnostic norms of gonadotropin responses to GnRH in this age group, including a luteinizing hormone (LH) response greater than in older children with central precocious puberty and a peak LH/follicle stimulating hormone (FSH) ratio higher than in infants without central precocious puberty.

THE USE OF GnRH ANALOGUES AS DIAGNOSTIC TESTS

There were two reports on the use of GnRHa for diagnostic testing. Kletter and colleagues [133] found a significant response of plasma gonadotropins to one single subcutaneous injection of GnRHa in boys with constitutional delay of growth and adolescence, in contrast to boys with hypogonadotropic hypogonadism who had no significant response. Thus, one single subcutaneous injection of GnRHa can distinguish between the two conditions, in contrast to the prolonged overnight hormonal estimation.

Metera and colleagues [131] (their study was submitted to but not presented at the Symposium) have found that the plasma gonadotropin response 30 and 120 min after the GnRHa depot injection correlates significantly with the respective gonadotropin response during the conventional GnRH test. They obtained with both methods a pubertal response in patients with gonadotropin-dependent precocious puberty, before gonadotropin suppression with the GnRHa was achieved, and a prepubertal response in treated patients, and in patients with gonadotropin-independent precocious puberty. Thus, one measurement of gonadotropins 120 min after GnRHa depot injection can be used as a reliable test for monitoring therapy and distinguishing between gonadotropin-dependent and gonadotropin-independent sexual precocity.

Following the encouraging results of GnRHa therapy on the final height of children with central precocious puberty, therapeutic trials were carried out with GnRHa in children with growth hormone deficiency as well as in normal early pubertal children with short stature, in an attempt to improve their final height, by suppressing pubertal development with the GnRHa and stimulating growth with growth hormone. According to earlier studies[56,58] on short-term follow-up, this combined therapy did not prove to be more effective as compared to growth hormone therapy alone.

GnRHa AS COMPLEMENTARY THERAPY TO GROWTH HORMONE THERAPY

Baens, Gschwend and Lee [130] reported a comparative study on patients with growth hormone deficiency associated with central precocious puberty. Two patients were treated with GnRHa alone, eight with growth hormone alone and 21 with a combination of the two drugs. The results revealed a better prognosis of final height for the patients treated with the combination of growth hormone and GnRHa.

A study on GnRHa therapy in combination with recombinant human growth hormone in normal pubertal short children (14 boys, five girls) was undertaken by Sack and Lunenfeld [134]. The aim of this study was to improve final height by accelerating growth while puberty is suppressed. It is of note that the growth velocity of the treated children was significantly increased, and during the period of the study (6–12 months) the bone age did not advance. It is too early to envisage the final outcome of this therapeutic regimen. As a trial to improve genetically predefined short stature, it will have important implications.

SUMMARY

(1) From the international experience on treatment of central precocious puberty with GnRHa so far, it can be concluded that there is a consensus that an effective and sustained suppression of gonadotropin secretion and of gonadarche is achieved by this therapy and that this suppression is fully reversible. There is also a consensus that the bone maturation rate decreases with this therapy and final height is improved. But there is still controversy on the extent of the benefit for final height, and a more conclusive consensus on that issue can be achieved with more data on patients who have completed their growth after therapy. For an objective evaluation of the achieved final height, it is of major importance to bear in mind the limitations of adult height predictions in abnormal puberty[61] and to take into consideration the genetic growth potential of each

patient. It is important to discourage in the patients' families unrealistic expectations of the effect of the therapy on final height and to explain to them that the aim of therapy in sexual precocity is to prevent loss from the adult stature which is genetically predetermined.

It is of note that the majority of the available long-term data on patients with central precocious puberty treated with GnRHa on girls, since central precocious puberty is much less frequent in boys. Some early and limited data, also presented at the 1st Symposium[61–64] [130,134] questioned the reversibility of the testicular changes induced by GnRHa in boys with central precocious puberty. Reassuring, but still limited, information on this issue was presented at the 2nd Symposium[65], but there was none presented at this 3rd Symposium. Therefore, an important task for the future is to obtain more long-term data on male patients with central precocious puberty treated with GnRHa.

(2) The GnRHa can be used also as diagnostic agents in distinguishing different forms of abnormal puberty – precocious as well as delayed – and in monitoring gonadotropin suppressive therapy.

(3) The effectiveness of GnRHa and growth hormone therapy in growth hormone-deficient and in normal small children has not been proven so far and more long-term data are needed for its evaluation.

More long-term follow-up data are needed regarding the future of the treated children, concerning fertility and mineral bone content. On both these issues, the preliminary data presented at this Symposium and from the latest literature are encouraging. It can be expected that more information on these and all other issues will be presented at the next Symposium in 1996.

REFERENCES

1. Kuperman, H. S. and Epstein, J. A. (1962). Medroxyprogesterone acetate in the treatment of constitutional isosexual precocity. *J. Clin. Endocrinol. Metab.*, **22**, 456–8

2. Cloutier, M. D. and Hales, A. B. (1970). Precocious puberty. *Adv. Pediatr.*, **17**, 126–38

3. Lee, P. A. (1981). Medroxyprogesterone – a therapy for sexual precocity in girls. *Am. J. Dis. Child.*, **135**, 443–5

4. Sherins, R. J., Gandy, H. N., Thorslund, T. V. and Paulsen, C. A. (1971). Pituitary and testicular function studies. 1. Experience with a new gonadal inhibitor

17-alfa-Pregn-4-en-20-yno-(3,3-d)isoxazol-17-ol (danazol). *J. Clin. Endocrinol. Metab.*, **32**, 522–31

5. Teller, W. M., Murset, G. and Schellong, G. (1969). Urinary C19 and C21 steroid patterns in isosexual precocious puberty during long term treatment with gestagens. *Acta Paediatr. Scand.*, **58**, 385–92

6. Helge, H., Weber, B., Hammerstein, I. and Neumann, F. (1969). Idiopathic precocious puberty, indications for use of cyproterone acetate, an antigonadotrophic and antiandrogenic substance? *Acta Paediatr. Scand.*, **58**, 672

7. Rager, K., Huenges, R., Gupta, D. and Bierrich, J. R. (1973). The treatment of precocious puberty with cyproterone acetate. *Acta Endocrinol.*, **74**, 399–408

8. Bossi, E., Zurrugg, R. P. and Joss, E. E. (1973). Improvement of adult height prognosis in precocious puberty by cyproterone acetate. *Acta Paediatr. Scand.*, **62**, 405–12

9. Kauli, R., Pertzelan, A., Prager-Lewin, R., Grunbaum, M. and Laron, Z. (1976). Cyproterone acetate in the treatment of precocious puberty. *Arch. Dis. Child.*, **51**, 202–8

10. Kauli, R. and Laron, Z. (1980). Pubertal development in girls with sexual precocity after discontinuation of treatment with cyproterone acetate. *Helv. Paediatr. Acta*, **35**, 149–54

11. Coy, D. H., Vilchez-Martinez, J. A., Coy, E. J. and Schally, A. V. (1976). Analogues of luteinizing hormone releasing hormone with increased biological activity produced by D-aminoacid substitutions in position 6. *J. Med. Chem.*, **19**, 423–5

12. Laron, Z., Dickerman, Z., Ben Zeev, Z., Prager-Lewin, R., Comaru-Schally, A. M. and Schally, A. V. (1981). Long term effect of D-TRP-6-LHRH on testicular size, LH, FSH, and testosterone levels in hypothalamic hypogonadotrophic males. *Fertil. Steril.*, **35**, 328–31

13. Crowley, W. F., Comite, F., Vale, W. W., Rivier, J., Loriaux, D. L. and Cutler, G. B. Jr. (1981). Therapeutic use of pituitary desensitization with acting LHRH agonist: a potential new treatment of idiopathic precocious puberty. *J. Clin. Endocrinol. Metab.*, **52**, 370–2

14. Laron, Z., Kauli, R., Ben-Zeev, Z., Comaru-Schally, A. M. and Schally, A. V. (1981). D-TRP-6-analogue of luteinizing hormone-releasing hormone in combination with cyproterone acetate to treat precocious puberty. *Lancet*, **1**, 955–66

15. Comite, F., Gordon, M. D., Cutler, G. B., Jr., River, J., Vale, W. W., Loriaux, D. L. and Crowley, W. F. Jr. (1981). Short-term treatment of idiopathic precocious puberty with long-acting analogue of luteinizing hormone-releasing hormone. *N. Engl. J. Med.*, **305**, 1545–50

16. Mansfield, M. J., Beardsworth, D. E., Loughlin, J. S., Crawford, J. D., Bode, H. H., Rivier, J., Vale, W. W., Kushner, D. C., Criegler, J. F. and Crowley, W. F. Jr. (1983). Long term treatment of central precocious puberty with a long-acting analogue of luteinizing hormone-releasing hormone. *N. Engl. J. Med.*, **309**, 1286–90

17. Comite, F., Cutler, G. B. Jr. and Loriaux, D. L. (1984). LHRH analogue therapy of precocious puberty. In Vickery, B. H. (ed.) *LHRH and its Analogues*, pp. 315–28. (Lancaster: MTP Press)

18. Holland, F. J., Fishman, L., Luder, A., Costigan, D. C., Jenner, M. R., Weilgosz, G. and Fasekas, A. T. A. (1984). Subcutaneous and intranasal D-Ser-(TBU)-6-EA 10-LHRH (Buserelin) in management of precocious puberty. In Labrier, F., Belanger, A. and Dupont, A. (eds.) *LHRH and its Analogues, Basal and Clinical Aspects*, pp. 407–23. (Amsterdam: Excerpta Medica)

19. Kauli, R., Pertzelan, A., Ben-Zeev, Z., Prager-Lewin, R., Kaufman, H., Comaru-Schally, A. M., Schally, A. V. and Laron, Z. (1984). Treatment of precocious puberty with LHRH analogue in combination with cyproterone acetate – further experience. *Clin. Endocrinol.*, **20**, 377–84

20. Luder, A. M., Holland, F. J., Costigan, D. C., Jenner, M. R., Weilgosz, G. and Fazekas, A. T. A. (1984). Intranasal and subcutaneous treatment of central precocious puberty in both sexes with a long-acting analogue of luteinizing hormone-releasing hormone. *J. Clin. Endocrinol. Metab.*, **58**, 996–72

21. Stanhope, R., Adams, J. and Brook, C. G. D. (1985). The treatment of central precocious puberty using an intranasal LHRH analogue (buserelin). *Clin. Endocrinol.*, **22**, 795–806

22. Brauner, R., Thibaud, E., Bischof, P. and Rappaport, R. (1985). Long-term results of GnRH analogue (buserelin) treatment in girls with central precocious puberty. *Acta Paediatr. Scand.*, **74**, 945–9

23. Donaldson, M. D. C., Stanhope R., Lee, T. J., Price, D. A. and Brook, C. G. D. (1985). Gonadotropin responses to GnRH in precocious puberty treated with GnRH analogue. *Clin. Endocrinol.*, **21**, 499–503

24. Ward, P. C., Ward, I., McNinch, A. W. and Savage, D. C. L. (1985). Reversible inhibition of central precocious puberty with long-acting GnRH analogue. *Arch. Dis. Childh.*, **60**, 872–4

25. Styne, D., Harris, D. A., Egli, C. A., Kaplan, S. L., Rivier, J., Vale, W. and Grumbach, M. M. (1985). Treatment of precocious puberty with a potent luteinizing hormone-releasing factor agonist: effect on growth, sexual maturation, pelvic sonography and the hypothalamo-pituitary-gonadal axis. *J. Clin. Endocrinol. Metab.*, **61**, 142–51

26. Brauner, R., Thibaud, E., Bishop, P., Sizonenko, P. C. and Rappaport, R. (1985). Long term results of GnRH analogue (Buserelin) treatment in girls with central precocious puberty. *Acta Paediatr. Scand.*, **74**, 945

27. Boepple, P., Mansfield, J. M., Wiederman, J. M., Rudin, C. P., Bode, H. H., Criegler, J. F. Jr., Crawford, J. D. and Crowley, W. F. Jr. (1986). Use of potent long-acting agonist of gonadotropin-releasing hormone in the treatment of precocious puberty. *Endocr. Rev.*, **7**, 24–33

28. Pescovitz, O. H., Comite, F., Hench, K., Bannes, K., McNemar, A., Foster, C., Kenigsberg, D., Loriaux, D. L. and Cutler, G. B. Jr. (1986). The NIH experience with precocious puberty: diagnostic subgroups and response to short-term luteinizing hormone-releasing hormone analogue therapy. *J. Pediatr.*, **108**, 54

29. Roger, M., Chaussain, J. L., Berlier, P., Bost, M., Canlorbe, P., Colle, M., Francois, R., Garandau, P., Lahlu, N., Morel, I. and Schally, A. V. (1986). Long-term treatment of male and female precocious puberty by periodic administration of a long-acting preparation of D-TRP-6-luteinizing hormone-releasing hormone microcapsules. *J. Clin. Endocrinol. Metab.*, **62**, 670–7

30. Wiederman, M. E., Beardsworth, D. E., Crawford, J. D., Crigler, J. F. Jr., Mansfield, M. J., Bode, H. H., Boepple, P. A., Kushner, D. C. and Crowley, W. F. Jr. (1986). Adrenarche and skeletal maturation during luteinizing hormone-releasing hormone agonist suppression of gonadarche. *J. Clin. Invest.*, **77**, 121–6

31. Lahlou, N., Roger, M., Chaussain, J. L., Feinstein, M. C., Sultan, C., Toublanc, J. E., Schally, A. V. and Scholler, R. (1987). Gonadotropin and alpha-subunit secretion during long term pituitary suppression by D-Trp-6-luteinizing hormone-releasing hormone microcapsules as treatment of precocious puberty. *J. Clin. Endocrinol. Metab.*, **65**, 946–53

32. Drop, S. L. S., Odine, R. J. H., Rouwe, C., Otten, B. J., Maasschalkerweerd, M. W., Van Gons, A., Bot, A., Meradji, M., de Jong, F. H. and Slijper, F. M. E. (1987). The effect of treatment with an LH-RH agonist (Buserelin) on gonadal activity, growth and bone maturation in children with central precocious puberty. *Eur. J. Pediatr.*, **146**, 272–8

33. Kauli, R., Schally, A. V. and Laron, Z. (1990). Long term experience with a superactive Gn-RH analog in the treatment of precocious puberty. In Vickery, H. and Lunenfeld, B. (eds.) *GnRH Analogues in Cancer and Human Reproduction*, Vol. 4, *Precocious Puberty, Contraception and Safety Issues*, pp. 43–52. (Dordrecht, Boston, London: Kluwer Academic Publishers)

34. Drop, S. L. S., Oostdijk, W., Odink, A. J. H., Partsch, C. -J., Hummelink, R. and Sippell, W. G. (1990). Effect of GnRH analogues on growth and bone maturation: a role for growth factors and adrenal androgens. In Vickery, H. and Lunenfeld, B. (eds.) *GnRH Analogues in Cancer and Human Reproduction*, Vol. 4, *Precocious Puberty, Contraception and Safety Issues*, pp. 53–60. (Dordrecht, Boston, London: Kluwer Academic Publishers)

35. Boepple, P. A., Mansfiels, M. J., Crawford, J. D., Crigler, J. F. Jr, Link, K., Blizzard, R. M. and Crowley, W. G. (1990). Growth patterns and skeletal maturation during sex steroid suppression and reactivation in central precocious puberty. In Vickery, J. and Lunenfeld, B. (eds.) *GnRH Analogues in Cancer and Human Reproduction*, Vol. 4, *Precocious Puberty, Contraception and Safety Issues*, pp. 61–74. (Dordrecht, Boston, London: Kluwer Academic Publishers)

36. Kaplan, S. L., Stephure, D., Knezvic, J. and Grumbach, M. M. (1990). Precocious puberty: pathophysiology and treatment. In Vickery, H. and Lunenfeld, B. (eds.) *GnRH Analogues in Cancer and Human Reproduction,* Vol. 4, *Precocious Puberty, Contraception and Safety Issues,* pp. 75–83. (Dordrecht, Boston, London: Kluwer Academic Publishers)

37. Roger, M., Lahlou, N., Chaussain, J. L., Fouprie, C., Francois, R., Toublanc, J. E., Scholler, R. and Schally, A. V. (1990). Effect of GnRH agonists on pituitary gonadotrophins: dissociated secretion of subunits in children with precocious puberty treated with (D-TRP-6)LHRH microcapsules. In Vickery, H. and Lunenfeld, B. (eds.) *GnRH Analogues in Cancer and Human Reproduction,* Vol. 4, *Precocious Puberty, Contraception and Safety Issues,* pp.85–98. (Dordrecht, Boston, London: Kluwer Academic Publishers)

38. Monasco, P. K., Pescovitz, O. H., Feuillan, P. P., Hench, K. D., Barnes, K. M., Jones, J., Hill, S. C., Loriaux, D. L. and Cutler, G. B. Jr. (1988). Resumption of puberty after long-term luteinizing hormone-releasing hormone agonist treatment of central precocious puberty. *J. Clin. Endocrinol. Metab.,* **67**, 368–72

39. Kaplan, S. (1990). True precocious puberty: treatment with GnRH-agonists. *Gynecol. Endocrinol.,* **4** (Suppl. 2), 102 (Abstr.)

40. Chaussain, J. L., Bost, M., Colle, M., Francois, R., Lecornu, M., Malpeuch, G., Mariani, R. and Roger, M. (1990). Evaluation of growth and bone maturation after discontinuation of long term GnRH therapy in girls with idiopathic precocious puberty. *Gynecol. Endocrinol.,* **4** (Suppl. 2), 102 (Abstr.)

41. Sippel, W. G., Partsch, C. J., Hummelink, R., Oosdijk, W., Odink, R. J. H. and Drop, S. L. S. (1990). Posttherapy effect of GnRH analogues in precocious puberty (Dutch–German multicenter study). *Gynecol. Endocrinol.,* **4** (Suppl. 2), Addendum (Abstr.)

42. Boepple, P. A. and Crowley, W. F. Jr. (1990). GnRH agonist (GnRHa) therapy of central precocious puberty (CPP): impact on long-term growth and reactivation of gonadarche post treatment. *Gynecol. Endocrinol.,* **4** (Suppl. 2), 103 (Abstr.)

43. Kauli, R., Kornreich, L. and Laron, Z. (1991). Final outcome in precocious puberty treated with GnRH analogue. In Lunenfeld, B. (ed.) *Advances in the Study of GnRH Analogues,* Vol. 4, *The Basic Science of GnRH Analogues,* pp. 147–56. (Carnforth, UK: Parthenon Publishing)

44. Roger, M., Lahlou, N., Berlier, P., Swaenepoel, C., Bost, M., Colle, M., Malpuech, G., Mariani, R. and Chaussain, J. L. (1990). Recovery of gonadotrope and gonadal function in girls after treatment of precocious puberty with D-TRP-6-GnRH (Decapeptyl). *Gynecol. Endocrinol.,* **4** (Suppl. 2), 106 (Abstr.)

45. Brauner, R., Malandry, F. and Rappaport, R. (1990). Factors influencing the effectiveness of LHRH analogue therapy in girls with idiopathic central precocious puberty. *Gynecol. Endocrinol.,* **4** (Suppl. 2), 101 (Abstr.)

46. Metera, M., Romer, T. E. and Majcher, A. (1991). Central precocious puberty: improvement of growth potential under treatment with decapeptyl depot. In Lunenfeld, B. (ed.) *Advances in the Study of GnRH Analogues,* Vol. 2, *The Basic Science of GnRH Analogues,* pp. 169–76. (Carnforth, UK: Parthenon Publishing)

47. Nizzoli, G., Pellegrini, G., Fasolato, V. and Chiumello, G. (1991). Statural growth follow-up in patients with central precocious puberty treated with LHRH analogues. In Lunenfeld, B. (ed.) *Advances in the Study of GnRH Analogues,* Vol. 2, *The Basic Science of GnRH Analogues,* pp. 177–80. (Carnforth, UK: Parthenon Publishing)

48. Tengattini, F., Pedroncelli, A., Montini, M., Pagani, M. D., Gianola, D., Cortesi, D., Gheraldi, F., Sileo, F. and Pagani, G. (1991). Triptorelin (D-Trp-6-LHRH) during long term treatment of precocious puberty. In Lunenfeld, B. (ed.) *Advances in the Study of GnRH Analogues,* Vol. 2, *The Basic Science of GnRH Analogues,* pp. 181–6. (Carnforth, UK: Parthenon Publishing)

49. Henzle, M. R., Goodpasture, J. C., Rosenfield, R. L., Kaplan, S. L., Kirkland, J. S., Lin, T. -H., Comite, F., Jones, K. L. and Kaufmann, S. (1991). Nafarelin in management of central precocious puberty. In Lunenfeld, B. (ed.) *Advances in the Study of GnRH Analogues,* Vol. 2, *The Basic Science of GnRH Analogues,* pp. 195–206 (Carnforth, UK: Parthenon Publishing)

50. Lee, P. A. (1991). GnRH analogue treatment of precocious puberty: basal and GnRH-stimulated LH and FSH levels by RIA and FIA. In Lunenfeld, B. (ed.) *Advances in the Study of GnRH Analogues,* Vol. 2, *The Basic Science of GnRH Analogues,* pp. 161–7. (Carnforth, UK: Parthenon Publishing)

51. Sizonenco, P. C. (1991). GnRH analogues in the management of precocious puberty. In Lunenfeld, B. and Insler, V. (eds.) *The Current Status of GnRH Analogues,* pp. 89–96. (Carnforth, UK: Parthenon Publishing)

52. Kauli, R., Kornreich, L. and Laron, Z. (1990). Pubertal development, growth and final height in girls with sexual precocity after therapy with the GnRH analogue D-TRP-6-LHRH. *Horm. Res.,* **33**, 11–17

53. Jay, N., Mansfield, J., Blizzard, R. M., Crowley, W. F. Jr., Schoenfeld, D., Rhubin, L. and Boepple, P. A. (1992). Ovulation and menstrual function of adolescent girls with central precocious puberty after therapy with gonadotropin-releasing hormone agonist. *J. Clin. Endocrinol. Metab.,* **75**, 890–4

54. Feuillan, P. P., Jones, J. K. and Cutler, G. B. (1990). Girls with GNRH analog-resistant forms of precocious puberty. *Gynecol. Endocrinol.,* **4** (Suppl. 2), 105 (Abstr.)

55. Holland, F. J. (1990). Familial precocious puberty (testotoxicosis): etiological mechanisms. *Gynecol. Endocrinol.,* **4** (Suppl. 2), 105 (Abstr.)

56. Dewailly, D., Boute, D., Lepeut, M., Racadot, P. and Fossati, P. (1990). Evaluation of the diagnostic usefulness of a GnRH agonist testing in delayed puberty. *Gynecol. Endocrinol.*, **4** (Suppl. 2), 110 (Abstr.)

57. Pierson, M., Leheup, B., Jeandel, C. and Gendrault, B. (1990). Is final height prediction increased by LH-RH agonist in adjunction to rhGH given to deficient children? *Gynecol. Endocrinol.*, **4** (Suppl. 2), 109 (Abstr.)

58. Bernasconi, S., Volta, C., Tondi, P., Ghizzoni, L., Salvioli, V., Alberini, A., Baldini, A., Lamboghini, A. and Carani, C. (1991). GnRH analogue treatment in children with short stature. In Lunenfeld, B. (ed.) *Advances in the Study of GnRH Analogues*, Vol.2, *The Basic Science of GnRH Analogues*, pp. 157–60. (Carnforth, UK: Parthenon Publishing)

59. Brauner, R. and Rappaport, R. (1990). Should all girls with central precocious puberty be treated by LHRH analogue? In Vickery, H. and Lunenfeld, B. (eds.) *GnRH Analogues in Cancer and Human Reproduction*, Vol. 4, *Precocious Puberty, Contraception and Safety Issues*, pp. 39–41. (Dordrecht, Boston, London: Kluwer Academic Publishers)

60. Foutura, M., Brauner, R., Prevot, C. and Rappaport, R. (1989). Precocious puberty in girls : early diagnosis of a slowly progressing variant. *Arch. Dis. Childh.*, **64**, 1170–6

61. Zachmann, M., Sobradillo, B., Frank, M., Frisch, H. and Prader, A. (1978). Bayley–Pinneau, Roche–Wainer–Thissen and Tanner height predictions in normal children and in patients with various pathologic conditions. *J. Pediatr.*, **93**, 749–55

62. Hadziselimovic, F., Senn, E. and Bandhauer, K. (1987). Effect of treatment with chronic gonadotropin releasing hormone agonist on human testis. *J. Urol.*, **138**, 1048–50

63. Hadziselimovic, F. (1990). Influence of buserelin on testicular tissue after long-term treatment for precocious puberty and prostatic cancer. In Vickery, H. and Lunenfeld, B. (eds.) *GnRH Analogues in Cancer and Human Reproduction*, Vol. 4, *Precocious Puberty, Contraception and Safety Issues*, pp. 107–14. (Dordrecht, Boston, London: Kluwer Academic Publishers)

64. Tze, W. J., Gilks, B., Kitson, H., Couch, R. M., Taylor, G. P. and Merat, P. (1990). Testicular changes in patients with buserelin for precocious puberty. In Vickery, H. and Lunenfeld, B. (eds.) *GnRH Analogues in Cancer and Human Reproduction*, Vol. 4, *Precocious Puberty, Contraception and Safety Issues*, pp. 99–105. (Dordrecht, Boston, London: Kluwer Academic Publishers)

65. Tze, W. J., Stewart, L. J., Taylor, G. P., Kitson, H. F. and Couch, R. M. (1991). Reversibility of testicular changes in patients receiving long-term treatment with the GnRH agonist buserelin for precocious puberty. In Lunenfeld, B. (ed.) *Advances in the Study of GnRH Analogues*, Vol. 2, *The Basic Science of GnRH Analogues*, pp. 187–93. (Carnforth, UK: Parthenon Publishing)

BIBLIOGRAPHY

Abstracts of relevant papers presented at the 3rd International Symposium on GnRH Analogues in Cancer and Human Reproduction

125. Long term results of treatment of GnRHa therapy in central precocious puberty: height, gonadal function, bone density. R. Baens, P. A. Lee, USA

126. Precocious puberty during infancy: diagnosis and GnRHa treatment. S. Gschwend, P. A. Lee, USA

129. Final height (FHt) of girls with central precocious puberty (CPP): untreated and treated with cyproterone acetate (CyA) or with GnRH analogue (GnRHA). R. Kauli, L. Kornreich, L. Lazar, Z. Laron, Israel

130. GnRH analogue and growth hormone therapy among patients with central precocious puberty and growth hormone deficiency. P. A. Lee, S. Gschwend, R. Baens, USA

131. Decapeptyl-depot test (DD test) and GnRH test in diagnosis and monitoring of the treatment of precocious puberty (PP). M. Metera, T. E. Romer, A. Majcher, Poland

133. GnRH analog (Nafarelin): a useful diagnostic agent for the distinction of constitutional growth delay from hypogonadotrophic hypogonadism. G. B. Kletter, A. Rolfes-Curl, J. C. Goodpasture, L. Scott, M. R. Henzl, I. Z. Beitins, USA

134. Combined treatment of GnRH analogue and rhGH in pubertal normal short children. J. Sack, B. Lunenfeld, Israel

7

GnRH agonists in prostate cancer

F. Labrie

INTRODUCTION

As much as the blockade of testicular androgen secretion by treatment with gonadotropin releasing hormones (GnRH) agonists was an unpredictable discovery[1,2], the world-wide use of these peptides to achieve medical castration in men for the treatment of prostate cancer has been exceptionally rapid. In fact, since the first administration of a GnRH agonist to a man suffering from prostate cancer 13 years ago[3], the only side-effects observed in hundreds of thousands of men treated have been limited to those known to be associated with reduced androgen secretion by the testes, namely hot flushes and decreased, or loss of, libido and sexual potency. Following the discovery of the potent antigonadal effects of GnRH agonists and the description of their mechanism of action by our laboratory[2,3], a significant improvement has been the development of controlled-release formulations of these peptides, thus greatly facilitating their administration and the compliance of the patients.

DISCOVERY OF THE CASTRATION EFFECT OF GnRH AGONISTS

From many points of view, the antigonadal effect of GnRH agonists is unique in medicine. Usually, when the structure of a natural compound such as GnRH is elucidated, the goal of organic chemists is to synthesize analogues which are more potent than the natural compound, in order to use such compounds at low doses in the treatment of diseases resulting from a deficiency of the natural compound. Thus, as soon as the structure of natural GnRH became known[4], many research efforts were devoted to the synthesis of superactive analogues of GnRH. As demonstrated by their luteinizing hormone (LH)-releasing activity in pituitary cells in culture as well as after single injection in laboratory animals, peptides having 100–400 times the activity of natural GnRH were rapidly obtained[5]. Unexpectedly, however, following chronic instead of single administration of a GnRH agonist, the surprising observation made was a decrease in testosterone secretion by the testes, accompanied by an atrophy of the prostate and accessory sex organs[1,2].

GnRH AGONISTS IN PROSTATE CANCER THERAPY

Since the standard treatment of prostate cancer during the last 40 years had been orchiectomy or medical castration with high doses of estrogens[6,7], the discovery of the antigonadal effects of GnRH agonists in the male rat immediately suggested to us the possibility of using GnRH agonists to achieve medical castration in men suffering from prostate cancer. Thus, in the first man treated with a GnRH agonist for prostate cancer, castration levels of serum testosterone were achieved 2 weeks after starting treatment[3]. Since then, all GnRH agonists commercially available world-wide have shown 100% efficacy in blocking testicular androgen secretion, and castration levels of serum testosterone are known to be maintained as long as treatment continues (Figures 1 and 2).

While surgical castration presents psychological problems for many patients, high doses of estrogens cause serious cardiovascular complications which can lead to death in 15% of patients during the first year of treatment[8]. Thus, when endocrine therapy of prostate cancer is indicated, it is now well recognized that the choice of treatment to eliminate testicular androgens is orchiectomy or medical castration, achieved with a GnRH agonist (Figure 2). The long-term effects of the two treatments on prostate cancer are superimposable [113,146]. On the other hand, the potentially harmful effects of the transient stimulation of testicular androgen secretion, observed during the first days of treatment with a GnRH agonist, are completely eliminated by simultaneous administration of a pure antiandrogen[9–11]. As mentioned later in more detail, the simultaneous use of a pure antiandrogen (Flutamide or one of its derivatives) not only eliminates the risks of disease flare at the start

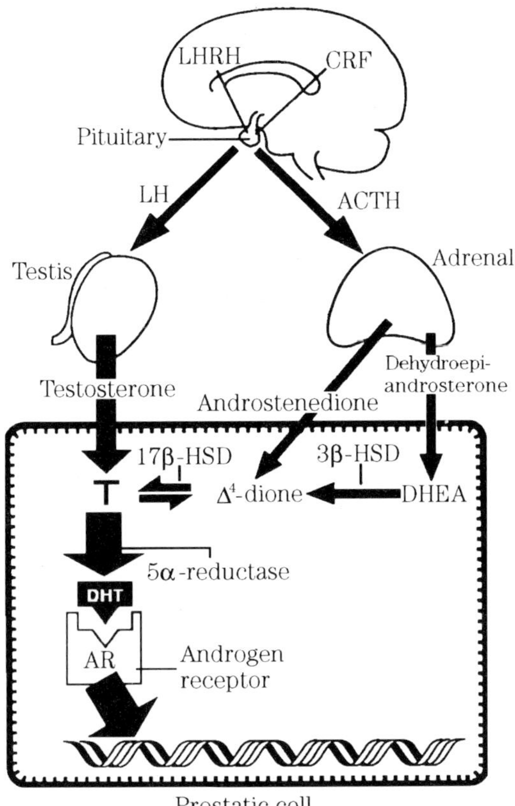

Figure 1 Intracrine activity of the human prostate or biosynthetic steps involved in the formation of the active androgen dihydrostestosterone (DHT) from testicular testosterone as well as from the adrenal precursors dehydroepiandrosterone (DHEA) and androstenedione (Δ^4-dione) in human prostatic tissue. 17β-HSD = 17β-hydroxysteroid dehydrogenase; 3β-HSD = 3β-hydroxysteroid dehydrogenase/Δ^5-Δ^4-isomerase. The widths of the arrows indicate the relative importance of the sources of DHT in the human prostate: 60% originating from the testes and 40% from the adrenals in 65-year-old men. The testis secretes testosterone (T) which is transformed into the more potent androgen dihydrotestosterone (DHT) by 5α-reductase in the prostate instead of secreting T or DHT directly, the adrenal secretes very large amounts of DHEA, while DHEA-sulfate (DHEA-S) and androstenedione (Δ^4-dione) which are transported in the blood to the prostate and other peripheral tissues. These inactive precursors are then transformed locally into the active androgens T and DHT. The enzymatic complexes 3β-HSD, 17β-HSD and 5α-reductase are all present in the prostatic cells, thus providing 40% of DHT

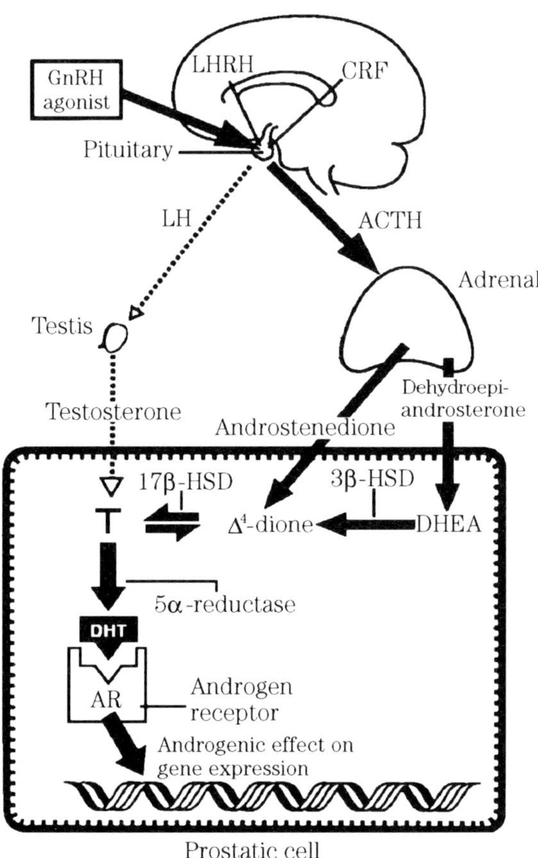

Figure 2 Schematic representation of the effect of treatment with a GnRH agonist on the androgens involved in prostate cancer growth. As can be seen by comparison with Figure 1, approximately 40% of DHT is left in the prostatic tissue following chemical castration with a GnRH agonist. The effect on prostate cancer is superimposable upon that obtained after orchiectomy

of treatment with the GnRH agonist but, most importantly, the antiandrogen neutralizes the action of the androgens of adrenal origin, which account for 40% of total androgens in men, and which are left free to stimulate prostate cancer after medical or surgical castration (Figures 2 and 3).

It is important to recognize that, although GnRH agonists offer a more acceptable method of castration free of the important side-effects of estro-

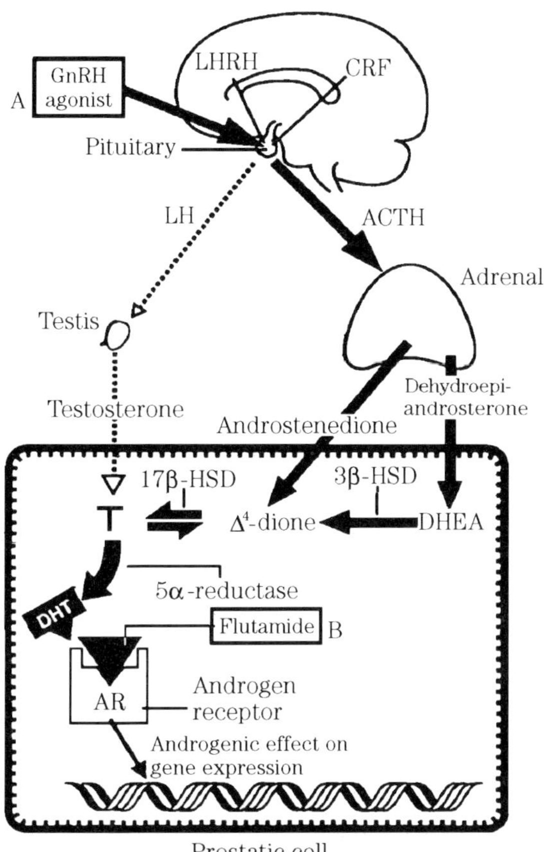

Figure 3   Schematic representation of the effect of combination therapy with a GnRH agonist and a pure antiandrogen (Flutamide) on prostate cancer growth. As can be seen in comparison with Figure 2, the antiandrogen blocks the access of DHT to the androgen receptor, thus greatly reducing the influence of androgens on genetic expression and prostate cancer cell growth

gens and of the psychological limitations of surgical castration, one cannot expect to improve the prognosis of prostate cancer beyond the results already achieved with orchiectomy[6,7]. In fact, GnRH agonists exert effects which are also limited to the blockade of testicular androgens. A recent study of the costs involved suggests comparable numbers for medical and surgical castration [109].

ADRENAL ANDROGENS ACCOUNT FOR 40% OF TOTAL ANDROGENS IN MEN

Following observation of the role of testicular androgens in prostate cancer in 1941[6], the most important discovery in the endocrinology of prostate cancer is the recognition that men are unique among animal species in having adrenals that secrete large amounts of the inactive precursor steroids dehydroepiandrosterone (DHEA), its sulfate (DHEA-S) and androstenedione (Δ^4-dione), which are converted into potent androgens in peripheral tissues, including the prostate (Figure 1). In fact, plasma DHEA-S levels in adult men are 100–500 times higher than those of testosterone[12], thus providing high levels of the substrates required for conversion into androgens in the prostate and other tissues. The local synthesis of active steroids in peripheral target tissues has been called intracrinology[13,14].

In order to stimulate prostatic growth, the adrenal steroid precursors, DHEA-S, DHEA and Δ^4-dione, must be taken up by the prostatic cells and be locally metabolized into active androgens (Figure 1). It has recently been demonstrated that the 3β-hydroxysteroid dehydrogenase, 17β-hydroxysteroid dehydrogenase and 5α-reductase genes are expressed in human prostatic tissue, thus providing the enzymatic machinery responsible for the high level of dihydrotestosterone formation in prostatic cells[14].

COMBINATION THERAPY WITH A PURE ANTIANDROGEN IS THE TREATMENT OF CHOICE IN ADVANCED PROSTATE CANCER

In order to take into account the role of both the testes and the adrenals in androgen formation in men, combination therapy was developed in order to block simultaneously both sources of androgens at the start of therapy in advanced prostate cancer[9,12]. The advantages of combination therapy have been confirmed by all four large-scale, double-blind and placebo-controlled randomized studies[15–17] [103–105,108]. In fact, these pivotal studies have demonstrated the important advantages of combination therapy, using a pure antiandrogen, on all the objective and subjective parameters studied. Of utmost importance is the observation that the simple addition of Flutamide added, on average 7.3[17] [104] and 15.0 [103] months of life, while the use of Anandron added 5.4[16] and 7.3[15] [105] months of life, respectively (Table 1).

Table 1 Combination therapy with a pure antiandrogen and castration in stage D_2 disease double-blind, randomized and prospective studies

	Number of patients	Best response	No response	Pain improvement	PSA or PAP normalization	Duration of response (months)	Death due to cancer (months)	Death from all causes (months)
NCI* Crawford et al.	602			$p < 0.05$	$p < 0.05$	16.9 vs. 13.8 (3.1 months) $p < 0.05$		35.6 vs. 28.3 (7.3 months) p < 0.05
EORTC[†] Denis et al.	307			$p < 0.05$	$p < 0.05$	16.4 vs. 10.6 (5.8 months) p = 0.002	48.0 vs. 33.0 (15.0 months) $p = 0.04$	38.1 vs. 28.8 (9.3 months) $p = 0.06$
Béland et al.[‡]	194	46% vs. 20% $p < 0.01$	20% vs. 38% $p < 0.01$	$p < 0.05$	$p < 0.05$	positive trend		24.3 vs. 18.9 (5.4 months) $p < 0.05$, n.s.
Janknegt et al.[†‡]	423	41% vs. 24% $p < 0.001$	22% vs. 36% $p = 0.002$	$p < 0.05$	$p < 0.05$	19.0 vs. 14.9 (4.1 months) $p = 0.006$	37.1 vs. 29.8 (7.3 months) $p = 0.041$	27.3 vs. 24.2 (4.1 months) n.s.

PSA, prostatic specific antigen; PAP, prostatic acid phosphatase; NCI, National Cancer Institute; EORTC, European Organization for Research and Treatment of Cancer

n.s., not significant, *Flutamide and gonadotropin releasing hormone (GnRH) agonist versus GnRH agonist as control; [†] Flutamide and LHRH agonist versus orchiectomy as control; [‡] Nilutamide and orchiectomy versus orchiectomy as control

In addition, the above-mentioned trials on combination therapy have illustrated the need to use large cohorts of patients in order to reach statistically significant differences in survival between the groups, thus indicating that many studies have too low a level of statistical power [107,110,112].

In three of the combination therapy studies[15,16] [103,105], the antiandrogen was added to the control arm at the time of progression. Such results clearly demonstrate the need to use combination therapy at the start of treatment, instead of at the time of relapse following failure of standard therapy. These observations argue extremely strongly against the suggestion of a two-step approach in the treatment of prostate cancer. With the knowledge of such data, it seems clear that combination therapy should always be applied as first-line therapy since, up to a large extent, the same treatment loses its efficacy when used as second-line therapy. This approach of maximal androgen blockade at the start of therapy is well supported by the accepted knowledge that patients relapsing after castration, estrogens or LHRH agonists have a poor or no response to adrenalectomy, hypophysectomy or Flutamide (see reference 12 for review). Moreover, strong support for the harmful effect of exposure of prostate cancer cells to low androgen levels comes from the recent observation that low serum testosterone levels are associated with shorter survival following androgen deprivation[18] [110]. In fact, low pretreatment serum testosterone levels before the start of endocrine therapy are associated with a poor prognosis, the significance of this variable being even more important than the extent of bone metastases [110]. These clinical data are well supported by our laboratory findings that low levels of androgens, comparable to those found after castration in men, induce the development of androgen hypersensitive tumors which are resistant to anti-hormonal therapy[19].

Such dramatic and negative effects of partial blockade of androgens, or low androgen levels which lead to shorter survival[15] [103,105] make unethical the use of any therapy having lower androgen-blocking capacity than the combination therapy using a pure antiandrogen in association with surgical or medical castration. It was thus judged unacceptable, by the participants at the Geneva meeting, to treat men suffering from prostate cancer with any treatment exerting a blockade of androgens inferior to that achieved by combination therapy using a pure antiandrogen and castration. The health regulatory agencies should thus use changes in serum testosterone levels to assess the efficacy of new GnRH agonists or new formulations of these compounds, instead of using survival as the parameter of response. It is, in fact, well recognized that men receiving a GnRH agonist alone will lose from 5.4 to 15.0 months of life[15,16] [103,105]. Such data also pose serious questions about the use of 5α-reductase inhibitors alone for the treatment of benign prostatic hyperplasia, knowing that a significant proportion of these men simultaneously have prostate cancer with could thus become resistant to endocrine therapy.

SERUM PSA IS A GOOD PREDICTOR OF LONG-TERM RESPONSE AND SURVIVAL FOLLOWING COMBINATION THERAPY

Measurement of serum prostatic specific antigen (PSA) has long been recognized as an excellent marker for the follow-up of prostate cancer patients treated by endocrine therapy as well as by surgery or radiotherapy. More recent data clearly indicate that measurement of serum PSA following endocrine therapy of advanced prostate cancer can be used as a predictor of disease-free survival as well as overall survival [104,105]. Since measurement of serum PSA is an objective and easily accessible parameter, it was suggested that measurement of serum PSA should be used as a parameter of response to assess the potential advantages of new treatments of prostate cancer. This approach would offer major savings and could well be more precise than the evaluation of clinical positive responses [108], while the use of survival as an endpoint is usually, if not always, complicated by the uncontrolled use of various therapies of unknown efficacy at the time of progression of the disease. The approval by government agencies of new drugs much needed for the treatment of prostate cancer could thus be accelerated markedly and costs would be significantly reduced.

MAJOR IMPORTANCE OF EARLY TREATMENT WITH COMBINATION THERAPY IN METASTATIC PROSTATE CANCER

An important observation made in all studies of stage D_2 patients, who received the combination therapy as initial treatment, is that prostate cancer is rapidly and extremely well controlled at the level of the prostate. Moreover, when progression of the disease occurs after an initial response, reappearance of the cancer takes place in the bones in approximately 98% of cases, while progression at the level of the prostate is rare (2% of cases). Such findings clearly indicate that the combination therapy is most efficient in blocking cancer growth at the level of the prostate, while the main problem is associated with tumors outside the prostatic area, usually in the bones. Such data strongly suggest that major efforts should be directed towards earlier treatment of the disease.

In order further to investigate the impact of 'early' versus late treatment in metastatic prostate cancer, we have stratified our cohort of stage D_2 prostate cancer patients according to the number of bone lesions. As illustrated in Figure 4, the median survival is not yet reached at 8 years in the group of patients having one to five bone metastases, while survival is dramatically reduced to 3.56 years when the number of bone lesions increases to between six and ten, thus representing a difference of more than 4.4 years. For the patients having 11–40 bone lesions, the calculated median survival was 2.36 years, while it was reduced to 1.76 years for those having disseminated disease or a superscan at the start of the same treatment.

It is thus clear from the present data that the addition of a relatively small number of bone lesions has a major negative impact on survival. It can also be seen in Figure 4 that, when the number of bone metastases goes beyond five, the increase in the number of metastases has less and less influence on the duration of survival under combination therapy, thus clearly demonstrating the major importance of not delaying treatment when the diagnosis of metastatic prostate cancer is made.

In agreement with these data, Crawford and colleagues [104] have reported that the patients having minimal disease display a much better response to combination therapy. In fact, recent analysis of the Intergroup National Cancer Institute study has shown an advantage of 19.5 months of survival for the patients with minimal disease who received the combination of leuprolide and Flutamide versus leuprolide and placebo, while the median overall survival of the whole group of patients was only 7.3 months. Similarly, in the European Organization for Research and Treatment of Cancer 30853 trial, combination therapy with Zoladex® and Flutamide, in patients having good (performance status 0–2, modest PSA elevation and T category < 4) or intermediate prognosis, led to a markedly improved disease-free survival as well as overall survival compared to the total group of patients [103].

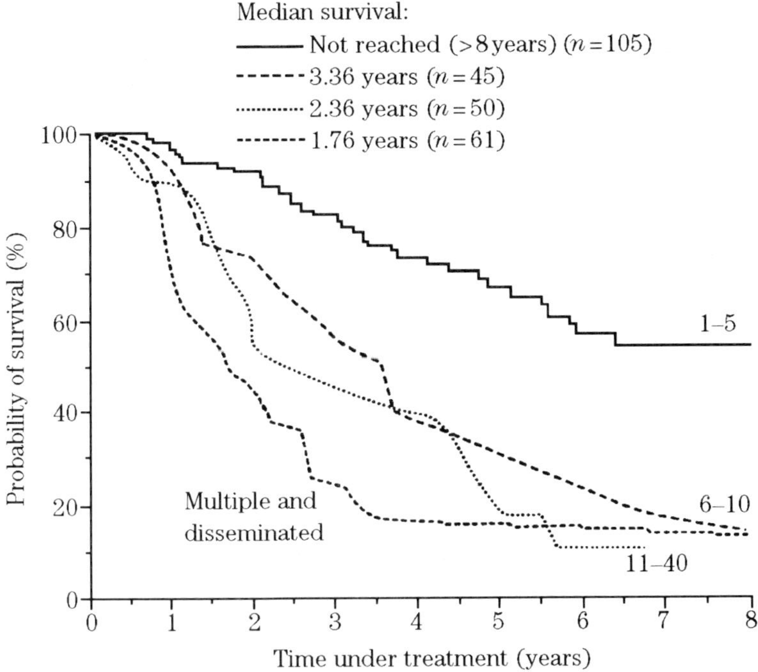

Figure 4 Probability of survival according to the number of bone metastases in previously untreated stage D2 prostate cancer patients who received the combination therapy with Flutamide and a GnRH agonist [D-Trp^6, des-Gly-NH$_2$^{10}]GnRH ethylamide

DOWNSTAGING OF LOCALIZED PROSTATE CANCER BY NEOADJUVANT THERAPY WITH FLUTAMIDE AND LUPRON

It is well recognized that the only opportunity for a curative therapy of prostate cancer is at an early stage when the disease is still localized to the prostate[20,21]. As well illustrated above, the limited potential for reducing mortality in advanced prostate cancer has stimulated major research efforts, in order to develop an efficient strategy for the diagnosis of early stage and curable prostate cancer[22,23]. Despite the recognized potential importance of early treatment, the wide acceptance of radical prostatectomy has been limited by the frequent finding that prostate cancer, presumed to be organ-confined at diagnosis, is found to be at a more advanced stage at histopathological analysis of the specimen following surgery.

Since recent studies have indicated that neoadjuvant combination therapy with the antiandrogen Flutamide and a GnRH agonist prior to radical prostatectomy[14,24–26] could decrease the incidence of cancer-positive surgical margins, we have performed a prospective and randomized study in order to assess the potential advantages of neoadjuvant therapy, with the antiandrogen Flutamide and the GnRH agonist Lupron®, on the incidence of positive margins at radical prostatectomy and on the histopathological stage of the cancer at surgery, compared with clinical staging at diagnosis.

Cancer-positive surgical margins were found in 38.5% (25/65) of control patients, while the incidence of positive margins was dramatically reduced to only 13.0% (10/77) ($p = 0.006$) in the group of patients who received the GnRH agonist and Flutamide for 3 months before radical prostatectomy (Table 2). Figure 5 shows that the decrease in cancer-positive surgical margins is of major amplitude at all stages of the disease except at stage B_0, where the number of patients was only two in each group. In fact, while positive margins were found in the surgical specimen in 15% of stage B_1, 35% of stage B_2, 55% of stage C_1, and 80% of stage C_2 control patients, the incidence of positive margins was decreased to 9% in stage B_1, 15% in stage B_2, 20% in stage C_1 and 17% in stage C_2 patients who received combination therapy for 3 months before surgery (Wilcoxon test, $p = 0.04$).

It is of special interest to see in Table 3 that the final stage determined following histopathological examination of the surgical specimen led to a 42.9% (33/77) improvement of the stage evaluated clinically at diagnosis in patients who received neoadjuvant combination therapy, compared to only 7.7% (5/65) in the control group. Upstaging (worsening of the stage), on the other hand, was seen in 61.5% (40/65) of patients who had radical prostatectomy alone. On the contrary, following 3 months of combination therapy, there was a dramatic decrease in upstaging from 61.5% to only 19.5% (15/77). While it was well recognized that combination therapy causes a decrease in

Table 2   Effect of 3-month neoadjuvant combination therapy with the antiandrogen Flutamide and the GnRH agonist Lupron on positive margins at radical prostatectomy in stage B and C prostate cancer

Group	*Negative margins*	*Positive margins*	*Total*
Control	40 (61.5%)	25 (38.5%)	65
Combination therapy	67 (87.0%)	10 (13.0%)	77
Total	107	35	142

χ^2, $p = 0.006$

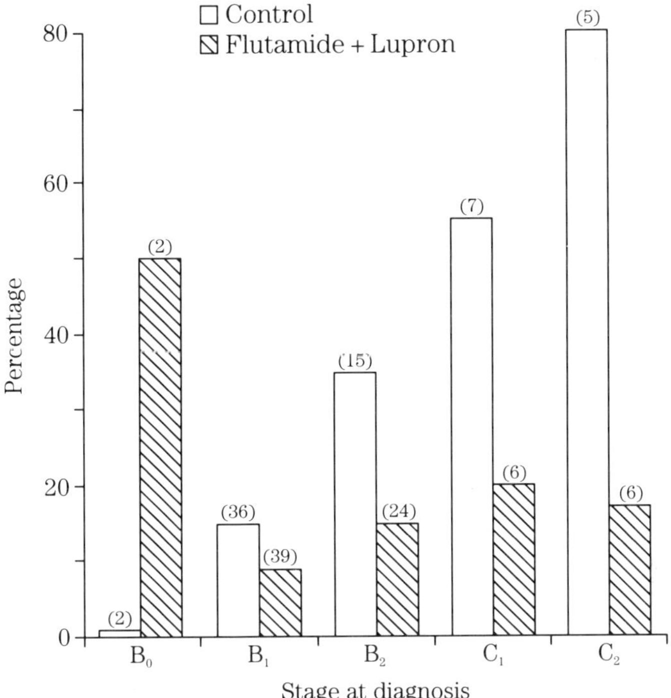

Figure 5 Effect of 3-month neoadjuvant combination therapy with Flutamide and Lupron on cancer-positive margins at radical prostatectomy at specific stages of prostate cancer, as determined clinically at diagnosis. The numbers in parentheses indicate the numbers of patients in each group

the total volume of the prostate, as well as a decrease in the volume of the cancer[14,24,25] [111], the present data show, in the first randomized clinical trial, that neoadjuvant combination therapy leads not only to downsizing but also to true downstaging of prostate cancer.

The present data thus demonstrate that neoadjuvant combination therapy improves the chance of having a favorable stage at surgery by 77.2%, compared to control patients not receiving the combination therapy. The main concern which has so far limited the acceptance of radical prostatectomy, namely a too optimistic evaluation of the stage of the disease at diagnosis, is thus dramatically improved by 3-month neoadjuvant treatment with Flutamide and a GnRH agonist.

An important aspect of the present approach is the use of a GnRH agonist in order to block temporarily the secretion of testicular androgens[3,10]. In fact,

Table 3 Effect of 3-month neoadjuvant therapy with Flutamide and a GnRH agonist on the histopathological stage of prostate cancer, compared to clinical stage at diagnosis

Group	B_0	B_1	B_2	C_1	C_2	Total
Downstaging						
Control	0% (0/2)	2.8% (1/36)	13.3% (2/15)	14.3% (1/7)	20.0% (1/5)	7.7% (5/65)
GnRH agonist + Flutamide	0% (0/2)	48.7% (19/39)	20.8% (5/24)	66.7% (4/6)	83.3% (5/6)	42.9% (33/77)
Upstaging						
Control	100% (2/2)	61.1% (22/36)	73.3% (11/15)	28.6% (2/7)	60.0% (3/5)	61.5% (40/65)
GnRH agonist + Flutamide	100% (2/2)	7.7% (3/39)	33.3% (8/24)	16.7% (1/6)	16.7% (1/6)	19.5% (15/77)
No change						
Control	0% (0/2)	36.1% (13/36)	13.3% (2/15)	57.1% (4/7)	20% (1/5)	30.8% (20/65)
GnRH agonist + Flutamide	0% (0/2)	43.6% (17/39)	45.8% (11/24)	16.7% (1/6)	0% (0/0)	37.7% (29/77)
Net change						
Control	+100% (2/2)	+58.3 (21/36)	+60.0% (9/15)	+14.3% (1/7)	+40.0% (2/5)	+53.8% (35/65)
GnRH agonist + Flutamide	+100% (2/2)	−41.0 (16/39)	+12.5% (3/24)	−50% (3/6)	−66.7% (4/6)	−23.4% (18/77)

while decreased libido and loss of sexual potency are observed in approximately 75% of patients treated with a GnRH agonist[12], return of libido and sexual potency is usually seen within a few months after cessation of treatment[14,24]. The GnRH agonist also prevents the potentially harmful effects of any increase in serum testosterone which could occur if a pure antiandrogen was used alone[12].

The success of the present approach relies, to a large extent, upon the availability of an efficient, low-cost and widely acceptable strategy to detect early-stage prostate cancer in the general population. In the randomly selected population of 7350 men examined at first visit, namely the Laval University Prostate Cancer Detection Program (LUPCDP)[23], 70.2% of the cancers discovered at first visit were at stage B, while 19.3% were at stage C and only 10.5% were at stage D. At 5781 follow-up visits, 82.4% of the cancers thus detected were at stage B and 17.6% were at stage C, while none was found at stage D[27] [106].

As shown in the present study, downstaging of prostate cancer with 3-month combination therapy dramatically improves the results of radical prostatectomy, thus giving the opportunity to 89% of patients, found as having prostate cancer at first visit, to become candidates for radical prostatectomy, and to nearly 100% of men, discovered as having prostate cancer at follow-up visits, to have access to the same potentially curative treatment. If annual or biennial serum PSA measurements are made, it is expected that more than 90% of the cancers detected will be candidates for radical prostatectomy, thus permitting, as demonstrated in the present study, to obtain negative surgical margins in 87% of cases or in approximately 80% of the total population of men who develop prostate cancer detectable by serum PSA and/or digital rectal examination.

Although the long-term effects of the present approach on survival remain to be determined by the follow-up of these patients, it is reasonable to expect that patients with localized disease at final histopathological staging, following radical prostatectomy, should have a life expectancy not different from that of men of similar age with no prostate cancer[20,21]. This is a complete reversal of the present situation where 75% of prostate cancers are already not confined to the prostate at diagnosis, and only prolongation of life can be offered to these patients by combination therapy.

MOST IMPORTANT POINTS OF GENERAL CONSENSUS MEETING

(1) Orchiectomy or treatment with GnRH agonists completely eliminates testicular androgens and has the same long-term effect on prostate cancer.

(2) Combination therapy with a pure antiandrogen (Flutamide or its analogue Nilutamide) in association with orchiectomy or medical castration (GnRH agonist) adds from 5.4 to 15.0 months of life in patients having metastatic stage D_2 prostate cancer.

(3) More years of life can be saved by treating with combination therapy stage D_2 patients having minimal disease or having one to five bone metastases, as compared to those having more advanced disease. Stage D_2 prostate cancer should be treated as soon as diagnosis is made since the disease is already very advanced.

(4) Combination therapy should be used as the reference endocrine therapy by regulatory agencies for comparison with new treatments of prostate cancer.

(5) Measurement of the efficacy of new GnRH agonists or new formulations of GnRH agonists should use serum testosterone as surrogate endpoint instead of positive clinical responses and survival. A pure antiandrogen should be given simultaneously with the GnRH agonist. Otherwise, months or even years of life are lost in the group of men who receive the standard treatment.

(6) Serum PSA should be used as surrogate endpoint for new endocrine therapies of prostate cancer.

(7) Major efforts should be made to detect and treat prostate cancer at an early stage. Moreover, investigations should be made to find the optimal duration of combination therapy before and after radical prostatectomy.

REFERENCES

1. Auclair, C., Kelly, P. A., Coy, D. H., Schally, A. V. and Labrie, F. (1977). Potent inhibitory activity of [D-Leu[6], des-Gly-NH$_2$[10]]LHRH ethylamide on LH/hCG and PRL testicular receptor levels in the rat. *Endocrinology*, **101**, 1890–3

2. Labrie, F., Auclair, C., Cusan, L., Kelly, P. A., Pelletier, G. and Ferland, L. (1978). Inhibitory effects of LHRH and its agonists on testicular gonadotropin receptors and spermatogenesis in the rat. In Hanson, V. (ed.) *5th Annual Workshop on the Testis: Endocrine Approach to Male Contraception. Int. J. Androl.*, Suppl. **2**, 303–18. (Scriptor Publisher APS)

3. Labrie, F., Bélanger, A., Cusan, L., Séguin, C., Pelletier, G., Kelly, P. A., Reeves, J. J., Lefebvre, F. A., Lemay, A. and Raynaud, J. P. (1980). Antifertility effects of LHRH agonists in the male. *J. Androl.*, **1**, 209–28

4. Matsuo, H., Baba, Y., Nair, R. M. G., Arimura, A. and Schally, A. V. (1971). Structure of porcine LH- and FSH-releasing hormone. I. The proposed amino acid sequence. *Biochem. Biophys. Res. Commun.*, **43**, 1334–7

5. Coy, D. H., Labrie, F., Savary, M., Coy, E. J. and Schally, A. V. (1975). LH-releasing activity of potent LHRH analogs *in vitro. Biochem. Biophys. Res. Commun.*, **67**, 576–82

6. Huggins, C. and Hodges, C. V. (1941). Studies of prostatic cancer. I. Effect of castration, estrogen and androgen injections on serum phosphatases in metastatic carcinoma of the prostate. *Cancer Res.*, **1**, 293–7

7. Veterans Administration Cooperative Urological Research Group (VACURG) (1967). Treatment and survival of patients with cancer of the prostate. *Surg. Gynecol. Obstet.*, **124**, 1011–17

8. Glashan, R. W. and Robinson, M. R. G. (1981). Cardiovascular complications in the treatment of prostatic carcinoma. *Br. J. Urol.*, **53**., 624–6

9. Labrie, F., Dupont, A., Bélanger, A., Cusan, L., Lacourcière, Y., Monfette, G., Laberge, J. G., Emond, J., Fazekas, A. T. A., Raynaud, J. P. and Husson, J. M. (1982). New hormonal therapy in prostatic carcinoma: combined treatment with an LHRH agonist and an antiandrogen. *J. Clin. Invest. Med.*, **5**, 267–75

10. Labrie, F., Dupont, A., Bélanger, A., St-Arnaud, R., Giguère, M., Lacourcière, Y., Emond, J. and Monfette, G. (1986). Treatment of prostate cancer with gonadotropin-releasing hormone agonists. *Endocr. Rev.*, **7**, 67–74

11. Labrie, F., Dupont, A., Bélanger, A. and Lachance, R. (1987). Flutamide eliminates the risk of disease flare in prostate cancer patients treated with an LHRH agonist. *J. Urol.*, **138**, 804–6

12. Labrie, F., Dupont, A. and Bélanger, A. (1985). Complete androgen blockade for the treatment of prostate cancer. In De Vita, V. T. Jr., Hellman, S. and Rosenberg, S. A. (eds.) *Important Advances in Oncology*, pp. 193–200. (Philadelphia: J. B. Lippincott)

13. Labrie, C., Bélanger, A. and Labrie, F. (1988). Androgenic activity of dehydroepiandrosterone and androstenedione in the rat ventral prostate. *Endocrinology*, **123**, 1412–17

14. Labrie, F. (1991). Endocrine therapy for prostate cancer. *Endocrinol. Metab. Clin. N. Am.*, **20**, 845–72

15. Janknegt, R. A., Abbou, C. C, Bartoletti, R., Berstein-Hahn, L., Bracken, B., Brisset, J. M., Calais da Silva, F., Chisholm, G., Crawford, E. D., Debruyne, F. M. J., Dijkman, G. C., Frick, J., Groedhals, L., Knonagel, H. and Venner, P. (1993). Orchiectomy and Nilutamide or placebo as treatment of metastatic prostatic cancer in a multinational double-blind randomized trail. *J. Urol.*, **149**, 77–83

16. Béland, G., Elhilali, M., Fradet, Y., Laroche, B., Ramsey, E. W., Trachtenberg, J., Venner, P. M. and Tewari, H. D. (1988). Total androgen blockade versus castration in metastatic cancer of the prostate. In Motta, M. and Serio, M. (eds.) *Hormonal Therapy of Prostatic Diseases: Basic and Clinical Aspects*, pp. 302–11 (Bussum: Medicom)

17. Crawford, D., Eisenberger, M. A., McLeod, D. G., Spaulding, J. T., Benson, R., Dorr, F. A., Blumenstein, B. A., Davis, M. A. and Goodman, P. I. (1989). A controlled trial of leuprolide with and without flutamide in prostatic carcinoma. *N. Engl. J. Med.*, **313**, 419–24

18. Soloway, M. S., Ishikawa, S., van der Zwaag, R. and Todd, B. (1989). Prognostic factors in patients with advanced prostate cancer. *Urology*, **33**, 53–6

19. Labrie, F., Veilleux, R. and Fournier, A. (1988). Low androgen levels induce the development of androgen hypersensitive cell clones in Shionogi mouse mammary carcinoma cells in culture. *J. Natl. Cancer Inst.*, **80**, 1138–47

20. Kolata, G. (1987). Prostate cancer consensus hampered by lack of data. *Science*, **236**, 1626–7

21. Brendler, C. B. and Walsh, P. C. (1992). The role of radical prostatectomy in the treatment of prostate cancer. *Cancer*, **42**, 212–22

22. Lee, F., Littrup, P. J., Torp-Pedersen, S. T., Mettlin, C., McHugh, T. A., Gray, J. M., Kumasaka, G. H. and McLeary, R. D. (1988). Prostate cancer: comparison of transrectal US and digital rectal examination for screening. *Radiology*, **168**, 389–94

23. Labrie, F., Dupont, A., Suburu, R., Cusan, L., Tremblay, M., Gomez, J. L. and Emond, J. (1992). Serum prostate specific antigen as prescreening test for prostate cancer. *J. Urol.*, **147**, 846–52

24. Monfette, G., Dupont, A. and Labrie, F. (1989). Temporary combination therapy with flutamide and Tryptex as adjuvant to radical prostatectomy for the treatment of early stage prostate cancer. In Labrie, F., Lee, F. and Dupont, A. (eds.) *Early Stage Prostate Cancer: Diagnosis and Choice of Therapy*, pp. 41–51 (New York: Excerpta Medica)

25. Solomon, M. H. (1990). Radical prostatectomy following androgen blockage. In Lee, F. and McLeary, R. L. (eds.) *5th International Symposium on Transrectal Ultrasound in the Diagnosis and Management of Prostate Cancer*, pp. 100–5. (Chicago: C. McAuley Health Center and Huron Valley Radiology)

26. Têtu, B., Srigley, J. R., Boivin, J. C., Dupont, A., Monfette, G., Pinault, S. and Labrie, F. (1991). Effect of combination endocrine therapy (LHRH agonist and

Flutamide) on normal prostate and prostatic adenocarcinoma: a histopathologic and immunohistochemical study. *Am. J. Surg. Pathol.*, **15**, 111–20

27. Labrie, F., Dupont, A., Suburu, E. R., Gomez, J. L., Cusan, L., Lemay, M., Koutsilieris, M. and Diamond, P. (1993). Serum prostatic specific antigen (PSA) is a highly efficient prescreening test for prostate cancer. Presented at *1993 Annual Meeting of the American Urological Association*, No. 12-733 (abst.)

BIBLIOGRAPHY

Abstracts of relevant papers presented at the 3rd International Symposium on GnRH Analogues in Cancer and Human Reproduction

103. Maximal androgen blockade-EORTC 30853 trial. C. Mahler, P. Whelan, L. Baert, A. Bono, D. Newling, L. Denis, Belgium

104. A comparison of Leuprolide and Flutamide vs Leuprolide alone in newly diagnosed stage D2 prostate cancer: Prognostic and therapeutic importance of the minimal disease subset. M. Eisenberger, E. D. Crawford, D. McLeod, R. Benson, A. Dorr, B. Blumenstein, USA

105. Long-term efficacy of maximal androgen blockade by Anandron combined with castration as first-line hormonal treatment of stage D prostate cancer reflected by early PSA normalization. R. Janknegt, The Netherlands

106. Advantages of neoadjuvant combination therapy with Flutamide and Lupron in early stage prostate cancer. F. Labrie, A. Dupont, R. Suburu, Y. Fradet, L. Cusan, J. L. Gomez, M. Lemay, B. Têtu, P. Diamond, Canada

107. Somatostatin analogue, BIM 23014 (Somatuline) and D-Trp-6-LHRH (Decapeptyl) in prostate cancer. H. Parmar, R. H. Phillips, S. Ghazali, I. W. H. Hanham, S. L. Lightman, UK

108. Progression in prostate cancer. D. W. W. Newling, The Netherlands

109. Cost–benefit analysis comparing D-Trp-6-LHRH (Decapeptyl) and orchiectomy in prostatic cancer. H. Parmar, R. H. Phillips, S. L. Lightman, UK

110. Zoladex with or without Flutamide in advanced prostate cancer: extended follow up and study of prognostic factors. R. O. Fourcade, P. Colombel, Ph. Mangin, P. Grise, J. Y. Soret, C. Coulange, G. Cariou, P. Coloby, M. Azab, France

111. Study of neo-adjuvant GnRH analogue Zoladex in locally advanced prostate cancer. R. O. Fourcade, P. Colombel, J. P. Sarramon, J. Toubol, M. Azab, France

112. LHRH analogues alone vs LHRH plus Flutamide in the treatment of advanced prostatic cancer. P. Ferrari, G. Castagnetti, G. Ferrari, C. A. Pollastri, Italy

113. Efficacy and safety of Leuprorelin acetate depot for prostate cancer in long-term follow-up study. D. Mulz, E. Kienle, G. Lubben, Germany

146. Buserelin 2 months implant (superfact depot) in the treatment of advanced prostatic cancer. R. Ackermann, L. Boccon-Gibod, B. O. Kihl, Sweden

8

GnRH analogues in the treatment of cancer of the breast and the reproductive organs

L. Kiesel

The proliferation of some gynecological tumors is sex hormone dependent and, therefore, the use of chemical agents that interfere with the hormonal milieu may provide a tool to regulate the growth of cancers of the breast, the ovary and the endometrium.

Gonadotropin releasing hormone (GnRH) analogues have been applied lately to patients with advanced stages of these carcinomas with variable success rates. Most experience has been achieved treating women suffering from mammary carcinoma, especially when metastatic disease was present. In some countries, GnRH analogues have already been approved for clinical use in breast cancer. More recently, the promising results obtained from the therapy of mammary cancer have stimulated trials using GnRH analogues for other malignancies in gynecology. The data for these indications are often preliminary, but have given insight into alternatives to established treatments.

BREAST CANCER

Breast cancer may affect approximately one in ten women in North America and Western Europe. The most effective way of managing the disease is early detection and surgical removal. Once the diagnosis of breast cancer has been made, it is essential to determine whether the disease is confined to the breast or whether it has disseminated to the regional lymph nodes or other sites. Since the presence and continued growth of metastases are the most common cause of death in breast cancer patients, great effort has been put into developing therapeutic regimens to prevent or to treat metastases.

Rationale for endocrine treatment

The growth of mammary carcinoma cells is promoted by a number of endocrine, autocrine and paracrine factors. For more than a century it has been known that oophorectomy will induce remissions in locally advanced disease[1]. This classical observation in premenopausal women has laid the foundation for the investigation and use of endocrine treatment.

During the past decades, various hormonal regimens have been applied to replace surgical palliative methods. Additive hormonal therapy was administered using antiestrogens, progestins and aromatase inhibitors.

Various factors are associated with the response rate of endocrine therapy. Estrogen receptor status and progesterone receptor status are the most effective prognostic tools. In addition, the site of metastases, patient age, menopausal status, disease-free interval as well as prior response to endocrine therapy are important predictors of response. The efficacy of the various endocrine therapies can be assessed by considering time to progression, and response rate.

The main *hormonal therapy* used in breast cancer is the antiestrogen tamoxifen. Given as an initial therapy, tamoxifen therapy is effective in 30–40% of patients with advanced disease. Their response rate of 30–35% has also been found with other endocrine regimens such as aminoglutethimide, hydrocortisone, estrogens, medroxyprogesterone acetate or megestrol acetate.

In an elaborate overview of the Early Breast Cancer Trialists' Collaborative Group in 1992[2], randomized treatment using tamoxifen has been analyzed in 30 000 women with early breast cancer. Adjuvant treatment with tamoxifen reduced recurrence-free survival and mortality significantly by 25% and 17%, respectively.

In general, side-effects of the treatment with tamoxifen are well tolerated (hot flushes, menstrual irregularities) or rare (rebound response and tumor flare). New antiestrogens (toremifene, droloxifene, trioxygene) are currently under investigation to provide even better efficacy.

Surgical ablative procedures such as oophorectomy, adrenalectomy and hypophysectomy have proved to be effective but were irreversible and involved considerable morbidity and mortality. The pharmacological effects of surgical castration also affect those patients that do not receive any clinical benefit from the operation. Since response rates are between 21 and 37%, a significant proportion of patients are also exposed to the risk of peri- and postoperative morbidity and mortality without the benefit of clinical response.

The effect of surgical ovariectomy can also be accomplished by using GnRH analogues to produce temporary suppression of estrogen serum levels via 'partial medical hypophysectomy' and 'reversible medical castration'. The main mechanism of action of the continuous treatment with GnRH analogues is most likely via the suppression of the neuroendocrine–ovarian axis. Recent reports of *in vitro* cell culture experiments and *in vivo* animal studies have provided some evidence that GnRH analogues may also provoke direct inhibition of breast cancer growth.

Clinical efficacy of the administration of GnRH analogues

The first studies of GnRH analogue treatment have been carried out in *premenopausal women* with metastatic breast cancer[3–8]. The average rate of objective response (complete or partial remission) following treatment with different types of GnRH analogues and different modes of their administration has been about 40% (range 30–60%). Stable disease was achieved in approximately 25–30% of cases. The disease-free interval was prolonged and the time to progression was dependent on the disease-free interval. In a large open phase II trial the overall response rate and duration following treatment with Zoladex® (goserelin) were related to an estrogen receptor-positive status[9].

The largest coordinated multicenter trial of the treatment of advanced breast cancer in pre- and postmenopausal women has been carried out using the monthly injection of Zoladex as an initial therapy in 333 women[10]. Efficacy data were analyzed from 228 eligible patients. At the time of entry to the studies, the majority (81.5%) had metastatic disease; the remaining 18.5% had advanced locoregional disease. Mean serum luteinizing hormone (LH) and estradiol concentrations were suppressed by day 22 after the first injection. Subjective response occurred in 68.3% of patients assessed. The median time to subjective response was 8 weeks (range 1–52 weeks). The objective response rate (complete and partial response) was 36.4% The median time to response among these patients was 12 weeks (range 4–49 weeks). The lifetable median duration of response was 44 weeks (range

4–160 weeks). Higher response rates were observed in the subgroups of women with tumors that were estrogen receptor-positive and those that were differentiated histologically, but responses were also achieved in estrogen receptor-negative and poorly differentiated tumors. In a small number of patients that have received previous hormonal therapy for advanced breast cancer, an overall objective response rate of 21.4% was achieved. Those patients that had not received hormonal treatment prior to Zoladex had a response rate of 37.4%. Objective response rate was independent of the premenopausal age of the patients investigated in this study.

Clinical efficacy of combined administration of GnRH analogues and other hormonal agents

A randomized trial is presently being performed to investigate the effect of Zoladex (goserelin) versus Zoladex plus Nolvadex® (tamoxifen) in 317 patients with advanced breast cancer in the UK. An interim analysis of this study presented by R. W. Blamey [114] showed no significant difference between the two groups regarding patients responding to therapy. Complete and partial remission was 32% in the Zoladex versus 38% in the Zoladex plus Nolvadex group. Overall time to progression, however, was significantly longer in patients treated with Zoladex plus Nolvadex (median 59 weeks in the Zoladex group versus 88 weeks in the Zoladex plus Nolvadex group). At present, there are no differences in the survival demonstrable between the groups.

Peripheral aromatization seems to be largely unaffected by GnRH agonist treatment, although the suppression of ovarian androgen synthesis reduces the plasma levels of substrate for aromatase. During GnRH agonist therapy, plasma estrogen levels are generally within the postmenopausal range, but in some patients partial recovery of follicular activity may occur. By the end of a 6-month course of GnRH agonist treatment, about 75% of patients had higher levels of serum estradiol than at the time of full suppression at week 4. A study with a small number of patients ($n = 6$) has investigated the inhibition of aromatization by 4-hydroxyandrostenedione (4-OHA) alone or in combination with Zoladex for the treatment of premenopausal breast cancer patients[11,12]. The combination of both drugs caused a greater estrogen suppression than Zoladex alone and led to objective clinical response in four out of six breast cancer patients after their relapse from treatment with Zoladex as a single agent. This publication indicates that this combination of

GnRH agonist and an aromatase inhibitor should be subjected to clinical trails.

Binding and direct action of GnRH analogues in breast carcinoma – different mechanisms of GnRH agonists

Reports showing that GnRH agonists can be effective in postmenopausal women with metastatic breast cancer indicate that GnRH analogues may also act via mechanisms independent of ovarian steroid hormone suppression[13–19]. Positive therapeutical results in postmenopausal patients, however, have not been confirmed in other publications[20,21].

Various *in vitro* and *in vivo* experimental studies investigated the binding of GnRH analogues to breast cancer tissue[22–28]. Low-affinity but also high-affinity binding sites have been demonstrated in membrane fractions prepared from mammary carcinoma tissue. There have also been reports showing a failure to detect GnRH receptors in human benign and malignant breast tissue as well in MCF-7 and MDA-MB-231 cancer cells[29–34].

Both agonists and antagonists of GnRH seem to regulate the proliferation of breast cancer cells in culture or cancer tissue in animal experiments[35–43]. Most publications show an inhibitory effect of GnRH analogues on cancer growth without the clear antagonistic action of GnRH antagonists when compared to agonists. Some actions of GnRH agonists may become evident in the presence of other molecules. In an *in vitro* study Pasqualini and colleagues [117] demonstrated the inhibition of estrone uptake in MCF-7 breast cancer cells following the combined treatment with Decapeptyl and heparin. Neither of the two drugs had an effect by themselves. This observation may be relevant for the control of estradiol in hormone-dependent breast cancer.

In a study comparing different GnRH agonists in breast cancer, the administration of the novel GnRH analogues, folligen and ovurelin-C, resulted in a time-dependent decrease in the size of the ovary-dependent mammary tumors induced by DMBA[44]. The effect was comparable to those achieved by Zoladex or by surgical castration. However, the mechanisms of action of folligen and the superactive GnRH analogues were different. In animals treated with folligen, normal follicular maturation and development of corpora lutea were observed. Although the concentration of the circulating estradiol was decreased by folligen, the extent of this decrease was not as pronounced as in the case of surgically castrated animals. These data indicate that folligen did not cause follicular atresia, as observed in other superanalogues of GnRH, but was an effective antitumor agent.

When folligen was compared with buserelin, both analogues inhibited the proliferation of MDA-MB-231 human breast cancer cell line[45]. Significant differences, however, were found in the signal transduction pathways activated by these analogues. The activity of tyrosine kinase, which is thought to mediate some fundamental signals of cellular growth control, was inhibited by buserelin and to a lesser extent by folligen. On the contrary, folligen was more potent than buserelin in translocating protein kinase C from the soluble to particulate fractions in MDA-MB-231 cancer cells. Inositol phosphate turnover a third signaling pathway, was also differently modulated by the two GnRH analogues. Labeling of phospholipids was increased significantly by folligen, whereas no effect was observed using buserelin. These results demonstrate, for the first time, that tyrosine kinases, phospholipid turnover pathway and protein kinase C can be directly involved in the antitumor action of GnRH analogues. It appears that not all GnRH agonists have the same mechanism of action regarding direct antitumor growth effects.

In vitro experiments demonstrate the interference of the GnRH antagonist SB-75 with insulin-like growth factor (IGF) autocrine/paracrine pathways [118]. Previous studies have shown the antiproliferative action of SB-75 on basal and estrogen-induced growth of mammary cells. The mitogenic effect of IGF-I is three times more potent than that of IGF-II and 30 times more potent than that of insulin. The GnRH antagonist significantly inhibited basal, estrogen- and IGF-induced cell growth. The GnRH agonist itself did not exert any effect and did not antagonize the action of SB-75. The authors assume that specific receptors recognizing the GnRH antagonist may be present which do not bind the GnRH agonist. SB-75 also inhibited the release of IGF-II and increased the level of IGF binding proteins, suggesting that inhibition of growth factor secretion or the binding of IGFs is important for the inhibition of cell growth.

Recently, cytotoxic analogues of GnRH have been synthesized and their binding to GnRH receptors analyzed[46,47]. GnRH agonists and antagonists with high binding affinity to human breast cancer cell membrane can serve as carriers for cytotoxic compounds and target the chemotherapeutic agents to the receptors of cancer tissues. Reduced-size GnRH analogues carrying various cytotoxic agents (anthraquinone derivatives, methotrexate and platinum complex) have been synthesized. The hybrid molecules had no GnRH agonistic activity *in vitro* or *in vivo* but had non-typical antagonistic effects on pituitary cells. These analogues showed a wide range of receptor-binding affinities to membranes of breast cancer. Several of these conjugates exerted some cytotoxic effects on the MCF-7 breast cancer cell line. Because the antitumor action of these cytotoxic analogues may be directed more selectively towards cells that have cell membrane receptors, the peripheral toxicity could be reduced.

OVARIAN CANCER

Ovarian cancer is the fourth most frequent cause of death from cancer in women. Approximately one woman in 70 will develop ovarian cancer in her lifetime and one woman in 100 will die of this cancer in the USA. A large number of women with ovarian cancer are already at an advanced stage of disease at the time of diagnosis. Optimal surgical procedure and postoperative chemotherapy for advanced ovarian cancer have been unsatisfactory until now. Alternative means of postoperative therapy with preferably less side-effects have been investigated.

For many years, hormonal regulation of the initiation and growth of ovarian cancer has been proposed in epidemiological studies. The protective effect of parity, multiple births, history of breast feeding and oral contraceptive use supports the 'incessant ovulation' hypothesis[48]. Women who have ever been pregnant or who have taken oral contraceptives have a 30–60% less chance of developing ovarian cancer than women without pregnancy or without oral contraception. Another explanation is proposed by the 'gonadotropin theory' whereby gonadotropins might promote the initiation and proliferation of ovarian carcinoma[49]. Cell growth of metastatic and *in situ* ovarian carcinomas is stimulated by the administration of gonadotropins[50,51]. Interestingly, estradiol had an inhibitory effect on cell proliferation.

The incidence of ovarian cancer increases during perimenopause in the presence of high levels of gonadotropins and a low serum concentration of estradiol[52]. Although LH and follicle stimulating hormone (FSH) receptors have been demonstrated in ovarian tumors, it is still unclear whether ovarian tumors are target tissues for gonadotropins.

Animal experiments have provided evidence for the stimulatory effect of gonadotropins on the development of ovarian cancer[53]. In W/W mice, goserelin injections prevented the development of ovarian complex tubular adenomas, possibly due to the suppression of elevated gonadotropin levels [117].

The administration of GnRH analogues could, therefore, exert a beneficial effect on ovarian cancer growth by suppressing gonadotropin levels or even prevent ovarian cancer[54].

Action and binding of GnRH analogues

As already described for breast cancer cells, a direct action of GnRH analogues on ovarian cancer cells has been suggested. Under experimental conditions, the growth of transplanted ovarian tumors in castrated rats was inhibited by D-Trp^6-GnRH[55]. Both agonistic and antagonistic analogues of GnRH directly inhibited the function or proliferation of ovarian cells in humans[56–58] [122].

Recently, the expression of GnRH was demonstrated in human ovarian cancer as a possible evidence for an autocrine regulation[59] [121]. Furthermore, immunoreactive GnRH was detected to be higher in human ovarian cancer than in normal human ovarian tissue. Extracts from ovarian cancers stimulated inositol phospholipid metabolism in an analogous manner to GnRH. It is, therefore, assumed that the chronic administration of GnRH analogues may induce desensitization of GnRH binding sites, thereby causing tumor regression.

Several authors have described and characterized binding sites for GnRH analogues in human ovarian tissue and carcinoma cells[60–62].

Clinical trials using GnRH analogues

Initial clinical trials have shown that the reduction of LH and FSH by (D-Trp^6)-GnRH can induce partial remission or lead to stable disease in patients with ovarian cancer relapsing after conventional treatment[63–69] [120, 122–124]. The administration of different types of GnRH analogues (triptorelin, leuprolide) resulted in partial remission or stable disease in 10–50% of patients with advanced ovarian cancer relapsing after conventional treatment. There was no correlation of response with histological subtype or grade, and there was no significant difference between the histology of the responding patients and the non-responding patients. Presently, a randomized prospective multicenter trail is being performed to investigate the efficacy of (D-Trp^6)-GnRH versus placebo, in addition to conventional surgery and chemotherapy in cases of ovarian cancer stages III and IV [122]. Preliminary results of this on-going study appear to support the previous findings of some benefit in complete and partial response. For the treatment of progressive ovarian cancer in patients in whom all other established treatment modalities have been exhausted, Decapeptyl was compared with tamoxifen in a randomized study [123]. In this study, the median survival time after randomization was 6 months without any significant difference between the two groups. The authors of that report propose the use of GnRH analogues under these circumstances since second-line chemotherapy did not provide better results.

ENDOMETRIAL CANCER

In the Western hemisphere, the incidence of endometrial cancer has been increasing during the past few decades. Hormonal therapy has been a part of conventional therapy in advanced and metastasized endometrial cancer. Good response rates have been achieved using high-dose progestin treatment, especially if the tumor is well differentiated and progesterone receptors are positive.

Recently, specific binding sites have been demonstrated in endometrial cancer tissues and cell lines[70] [122]. These and other observations led to trials to investigate the efficacy of GnRH analogues in women with recurrent endometrial cancer[71]. In this study, 17 patients with symptomatic, progressive and measurable disease were treated with GnRH analogues (leuprolide or goserelin). All patients had received earlier treatment with progestins. A response was achieved in six out of 17 patients (35%) with one complete and five partial remissions. Radiotherapy and medroxyprogesterone acetate had failed in all the responders. Although experience with GnRH agonists is very limited in endometrial cancer, further studies should try to confirm the antiproliferative action of these analogues in patients with endometrial cancer.

REFERENCES

1. Beatson, G. T. (1986). On the treatment of inoperable cases of carcinoma of the mamma: suggestions for a new method of treatment with illustrative cases. *Lancet*, **2**, 104

2. Early Breast Cancer Trialists' Collaborative Group (1992). Systemic treatment of early breast cancer by hormonal, cytotoxic, or immune therapy. *Lancet*, **339**, 1–15

3. Klijn, J. G. M. and De Jong, F. H. (1982). Treatment with a luteinizing-hormone releasing-hormone analogue (buserelin) in premenopausal patients with metastatic breast cancer. *Lancet.* **1**, 1213–16

4. Klijn, J. G. M., De Jong, F. H., Blankenstein, M. A., Docter, R., Alexieva-Figusch, J., Blonk-van der Wijst, J., Lamberts, S. W. J. (1984). Anti-tumor and endocrine effects of chronic LHRH agonist (buserelin) treatment with or without tamoxifen in premenopausal metastatic breast cancer. *Breast Cancer Res. Treatm.*, **4**, 209–20

5. Harvey, H. A., Lipton, A., Max, D. T., Pearlman, H. G., Diaz-Perches, R. and de la Garza, J. (1985). Medical castration produced by the GnRH analogue leuprolide to treat metastatic breast cancer. *J. Clin. Oncol.*, **3**, 1068–72

6. Höffken, K. Miller, B., Fischer, P., Becker, R., Kurschel, E., Scheulen, M. E., Miller, A. A., Callies, R. and Schmidt, O. G. (1986). Buserelin in treatment of premenopausal advanced breast cancer. *Eur. J. Cancer Clin. Oncol.*, **22**, 746

7. Walker, K. J., Turkes, A., Williams, M., Blamey, R. W. and Nicholson, R. I. (1986). Preliminary endocrinological evaluation of sustained-release formulation of the LH-releasing hormone agonist D-Ser $(Bu^t)^6$ Azgly^{10} LH-RH in premenopausal women with advanced breast cancer. *J. Endocrinol.*, **111**, 349–53

8. Kaufmann, M., Schmid, H., Kiesel, L. and Klinga, K. (1989). GnRH-Agonisten (Zoladex)-Therapie bei prämenopausalen Frauen mit metastasierendem Mammakarzinom. *Geburtshilfe Frauenheilkd.*, **49**, 611–17

9. Kaufmann, M., Jonat, W., Kleeberg, U., Eiermann, W., Jänicke, F., Hilfrich, J., Kreienberg, R., Albrecht, M., Weitzel, H-K., Schmidt, H., Strünz, P., Schachner-Wünschmann, E., Bastert, G. and Maas, H. (1989). Goserelin, a depot gonadotrophin-releasing hormone agonist in the treatment of premenopausal patients with metastatic breast cancer. *J. Clin. Oncol.*, **7**, 1113–19

10. Blamey, R. W., Jonat, W., Kaufmann, M., Raffaello Bianco, A. and Namer, M. (1992). Goserelin depot in the treatment of premenopausal advanced breast cancer. *Eur. J. Cancer*, **28A**, 810–14

11. Stein, R. C., Dowsett, M., Hedley, A., Gazet, J. -C., Ford, H. T. and Coombes, R. C. (1990). The clinical and endocrine effects of 4-hydroxyandrostenedione alone and in combination with goserelin in premenopausal women with advanced breast cancer. *Br. J. Cancer*, **62**, 679–83

12. Dowsett, M., Stein, R. C. and Coombes, R. C. (1992). Aromatization inhibition alone or in combination with GnRH agonists for the treatment of premenopausal breast cancer patients. *J. Steroid Biochem. Mol. Biol.*, **43**, 155–9

13. Harvey, H. A., Lipton, A., Santen, R. J., Escher, G. C., Hardy, M. N., Glode, I. M., Segaloff, A., Landau, R. Z., Schneir, H. and Max, D. T. (1981). Phase II study of a

gonadotropin-releasing hormone analogue (leuprolide) in postmenopausal advanced breast cancer patients. *Proc. Am. Assoc. Cancer Res./Am. Soc. Clin. Oncol.*, **22**, 444 (Abstr.)

14. Waxman, J. H., Harland, S. J., Coombes, R. C., Wrigley, P. F. M., Malpas, J. S., Powles, T. and Lister, T. A. (1985). The treatment of postmenopausal women with advanced breast cancer with buserelin. *Cancer Chemother. Pharmacol.*, **15**, 171–3

15. Plowman, P. N., Nicholson, R. I. and Walker, K. J. (1986). Remission of postmenopausal breast cancer during treatment with the luteinizing hormone releasing hormone agonist ICI 118630. *Br. J. Cancer*, **54**, 903–9

16. Schwartz, L., Guiochet, N. and Keiling, R. (1988). Two partial remissions induced by an LHRH analogue in two postmenopausal women with metastatic breast cancer. *Cancer*, **62**, 2498–500

17. Cassano, A., Astone, A., Garufi, C. Noviello, M. R., Pietrantonio, F. and Barone, C. (1989). A response in advanced post-menopausal breast cancer during treatment with the luteinising hormone releasing hormone agonist Zoladex. *Cancer Lett.*, **48**, 123–4

18. Crighton, I. L., Dowsett, M., Lal, A., Man, A. and Smith, I. E. (1989). Use of luteinising hormone-releasing hormone agonist (Leuprorelin) in advanced post-menopausal breast cancer: clinical and endocrine effects. *Br. J. Cancer*, **60**, 644–8

19. Harris, A. L., Carmichael, J., Cantwell, B. M. J. and Dowsett, M. (1989). Zoladex: endocrine and therapeutic effects in post-menopausal breast cancer. *Br. J. Cancer*, **59**, 97–9

20. Wilding, G., Cehn, M. and Gelmann, E. P. (1987). LHRH agonists and human breast cancer cells. *Nature (London)*, **329**, 770

21. Slotman, B. J., Poels, L. G. and Rao, B. R. (1989). A direct LHRH-agonist action on cancer cells is unlikely to be the cause of response to LHRH-agonist treatment. *Anticancer Res.*, **9**, 77–80

22. Eidne, K. A., Flanagan, C. A., Harris, N. S. and Millar, R. P. (1987). Gonadotropin-releasing hormone (GnRH)-binding sites in human breast cancer cell lines and inhibitory effects of GnRH antagonists. *J. Clin. Endocrinol. Metab.*, **64**, 425–32

23. Eidne, K. A., Flanagan, C. A. and Millar, P. (1985). Gonadotropin-releasing hormone binding sites in human breast carcinoma. *Science*, **9**, 989–91

24. Kiesel, L., Kaufmann, M., Haeseler, F., Klinga, K., von Holst, T., Schmidt, W. and Runnebaum, B. (1988). GnRH-Rezeptoren im menschlichen Mammakarzinomgewebe. *Geburtshilfe Frauenheilk.*, **48**, 420–4

25. Fekete, M., Wittliff, J. L. and Schally, A. V. (1989). Characteristics and distribution of receptors for [D-Trp^6]-luteinizing hormone-releasing hormone, somatostatin, epidermal growth factor, and sex steroids in 500 biopsy samples of human breast cancer. *J. Clin. Lab. Anal.*, **3**, 137–47

26. Fekete, M., Bajusz, S., Groot, K., Csernus, V. J. and Schally, A. V. (1989). Comparison of different agonists and antagonists of luteinizing hormone-releasing hormone for receptor-binding ability to rat pituitary and human breast cancer membranes. *Endocrinology*, **124**, 946–55

27. Srkalovic, G., Szende, B., Redding, T. W., Groot, K. and Schally, A. A. (1989). Receptors for D-Trp^6-luteinizing horomone-releasing hormone, somatostatin, and insulin-like growth factor I in MXT mouse mammary carcinoma. *Proc. Soc. Exp. Biol. Med.*, **192**, 209–18

28. Baumann, K., Kiesel, L., Kaufmann, M., Bastert, B. and Runnebaum, B. (1993). Characterization of binding sites for a GnRH-agonist (buserelin) in human breast cancer biopsies and their distribution in relation to tumor parameters. *Breast Cancer Res. Treatm.*, **25**, 37–46

29. Mullen, P., Bramley, T. A., Menzies, G. and Miller, B. (1993). Failure to detect gonadotropin-releasing hormone receptors in human benign and malignant tissue and in MCF-7 and MDA-MB-231 cancer cells. *Eur. J. Cancer*, **29A**, 248–52

30. Seppälä, M. and Wahlström, T. (1980). Identification of luteinizing hormone-releasing factor and alpha subunit of glycoprotein hormones in ductal carcinoma of the mammary gland. *Int. J. Cancer*, **26**, 267–8

31. Sarda, A. K. and Nair, R. M. G. (1981). Elevated levels of LRH in human milk. *J. Clin. Endocrinol. Metab.*, **52**, 826–8

32. Bützow, R., Huhtaniemi, I., Clayton, R., Wahlström, T., Andersson, L. C. and Seppälä, M. (1987). Cultured mammary carcinoma cells contain gonadotropin-releasing hormone-like immunoreactivity, GnRH binding sites and chorionic gonadotropin. *Int. J. Cancer*, **39**, 498–501

33. Li, C. H., Ramasharma, K., Yamashiro, D. and Chung, D. (1987). Gonadotropin-releasing peptide from human follicular fluid. Isolation, characterization and chemical synthesis. *Proc. Natl. Acad. Sci. USA*, **84**, 959–62

34. Ciocca, D. R., Puy, L. A., Fasoli, L. C., Tello, O., Aznar, J. C., Gago, F. E., Papa, S. I. and Sonego, R. (1990). Corticotropin-releasing hormone, luteinizing hormone-releasing hormone, growth hormone-releasing hormone, and somatostatin-like immunoreactivities in biopsies from breast cancer patients. *Breast Cancer Res. Treatm.*, **15**, 175–84

35. DeSombre, E. R., Johnson, E. S. and White, W. F. (1976). Regression of rat mammary tumors effected by a gonadoliberin analog. *Cancer Res.*, **36**, 3833

36. Johnson, E. S., Seely, J. H. and White, W. F. (1976). Endocrine-dependent rat mammary tumor regression: use of a gonadotropin releasing hormone analog. *Science*, **194**, 329

37. Redding, T. W. and Schally, A. V. (1983). Inhibition of mammary tumor growth in rats and mice by administration of agonistic and antagonistic analogs of luteinizing hormone-releasing hormone. *Proc. Natl. Acad. Sci. USA*, **80**, 1459–62

38. Miller, R., Scott, W. N., Morris, R., Fraser, H. M. and Sharpe, R. M. (1985). Growth of human breast cancer cells inhibited by a luteinizing hormone-releasing hormone agonist. *Nature (London)*, **313**, 231–3

39. Blankenstein, M. A., Henkelman, M. S. and Klijn, J. G. M. (1985). Direct inhibitory effect of a luteinizing hormone-releasing horomone agonist on MCF-7 human breast cancer cells. *Eur. J. Cancer Clin. Oncol.*, **21**, 1493–9

40. Foekens, J. A., Henkelman, M. S., Bolt-de Vreis, J., Portengen, H., Fukkink, J. F. and Klijn, J. G. M. (1987). Direct effects of LHRH analogs on breast and prostatic tumor cells. In Klijn J. G. M. (eds.) *Hormonal Manipulation of Cancer: Peptides, Growth Factors and New (Anti)Steroidal Agents.* (New York: Raven Press)

41. Scambia, G., Oanici, P. B., Baiocchi, G., Perrone, L., Gaggini, C., Iacobelli, S. and Mancuso, S. (1988). Growth inhibitory effect of LH-RH analogs on human breast cancer cells. *Anticancer Res.*, **8**, 187–90

42. Sharoni, Y., Bosin, E., Miinster, A., Levy, J. and Schally, A. V. (1989). Inhibition of growth of human mammary tumor cells by potent antagonists of luteinizing hormone-releasing hormone. *Proc. Natl. Acad. Sci. USA*, **86**, 1648–51

43. Neri, C., Blangy, D., Schatz, B., Drieu, K., Berebbi, M. and Martin, P. -M. (1990). Direct inhibiting effect of (D-Trp^6) gonadotropin-releasing hormone on the estrogen-sensitive progression of polyoma virus-induced mammary tumors in athymic mice. *Cancer Res.*, **50**, 5892–7

44. Nicholson, R. I. and Kéri, Gy. (1992). Antitumor activity of Folligien, a novel gonadotropin-releasing hormone analogue against DMBA-induced tumors in the rat. *Tumor Biol.*, **13**, 44–50

45. Kéri, Gy., Balogh, A., Szöke, B., Teplán, I. and Csuka, O. (1991). Gonadotropin-releasing hormone analogues inhibit cell proliferation and activate signal transuction pathways in MDA-MB-231 human breast cancer cell line. *Tumor Biol.*, **12**, 61–7

46. Janáky, T., Juhász, A., Rékási, Z. Serfözö, P., Pinski, J., Bosker, L., Srkalovic, G. G., Milovanovic, S., Redding, T. W., Halmos, G., Nagy, A. and Schally, A. V. (1992). Short-chain analogs of luteinizing hormone-releasing hormone containing cytotoxic moieties. *Proc. Natl. Acad. Sci. USA*, **89**, 10203–7

47. Milovanovic, S. R., Radulovic, S. and Schally, A. V. (1992). Evaluation and binding of cytotoxic analogs of luteinizing hormone-releasing hormone to breast cancer and mouse MXT mammary tumor. *Breast Cancer Res. Treatm.*, **24**, 147–58

48. Fathalla, M. F. (1971). Incessant ovulation – a factor in ovarian neoplasia. *Lancet*, **2**, 163

49. McGowan, L. (1989). Epidemiology of ovarian cancer. *Oncology*, **46**, 51–62

50. Simon, W. E., Albrecht, M., Hansel, M., Dietel, M. and Hölzel, F. (1983). Cell lines derived from human ovarian carcinomas: growth stimulation by gonadotropic and steroid hormones. *J. Natl. Cancer Inst.*, **70**, 839–45

51. Wilamasena, J., Dostal, R. and Meehan, D. (1992). Gonadotropins, estradiol and growth factors regulate epithelial ovarian cancer growth. *Gynecol. Oncol.*, **46**, 345–50

52. Cramer, D. W., Hutchinson, G. B., Welch, W. R., Scully, R. E. and Ryan, K. J. (1983). Determinants of ovarian cancer risk. II. Inferences regarding pathogenesis. *J. Natl. Cancer Inst.*, **71**, 717–21

53. Peterson, C. M. and Ziminski, S. J. (1990). A long-acting gonadotropin-releasing hormone agonist inhibits the growth of a human ovarian epithelial carcinoma (BG-1) heterotransplanted in the nude mouse. *Obstet. Gynecol.*, **76**, 264

54. Pike, M. C., Ross, R. K., Lobo, R. A., Key, T. J. A., Potts, M. and Henderson, B. E. (1989). LHRH agonists and the prevention of breast and ovarian cancer. *Br. J. Cancer*, **60**, 142–8

55. Kullander, S., Rausing, A. and Schally, A. V. (1987). LHRH agonist treatment in ovarian cancer. In Klijn, J. G. M. (ed.) *Hormonal Manipulation of Cancer: Peptides, Growth Factors, and New (Anti)Steroidal Agents*, pp. 353–6. (New York: Raven Press)

56. Lamberts, S. W. J., Timmers, J. M., Osterom, R., Verleun, T., Rommerts, F. G. and De-Jong, F. H. (1982). Testosterone secretion by cultured arrhenoblastoma cells: suppression by a luteinizing hormone-releasing hormone agonist. *J. Clin. Endocrinol. Metab.*, **54**, 450–4

57. Tureck, R. W., Mastroianni, L. Jr., Blasco, L. and Strauß, J. F. (1982). III. Inhibition of human granulosa cell progesterone secretion by a gonadotropin releasing hormone agonist. *J. Clin. Endocrinol. Metab.*, **54**, 1078–80

58. Maruo. T., Otani, T. and Mochizuki, M. (1985). Antigonadotropic actions of GnRH agonist on ovarian cells *in vivo* and *in vitro*. *J. Steroid Biochem.*, **23**, 765–70

59. Aten, R. F., Polan, M. L., Bayless, R. and Behrman, H. R. (1987). A gonadotropin-releasing hormone (GnRH)-like protein in human ovaries: similarity to the GnRH-like ovarian protein of the rat. *J. Clin. Endocrinol. Metab.*, **64**, 1288–93

60. Bramley, T. A., Menzies, G. S. and Baird, D. T. (1985). Specific binding of a gonadotrophin releasing hormone and an agonist to human corpus luteum homogenates: characterization, properties, and luteal phase levels. *J. Clin. Endocrinol. Metab.*, **61**, 834–41

61. Pahwa, G. S., Vollmer, G., Knuppen, R. and Emons, G. (1989). Photoaffinity labelling of gonadotropin releasing hormone binding sites in human epithelial ovarian carcinomata. *Biochem. Biophys. Res. Commun.*, **161**, 1086–92

62. Emons, G., Pahwa, G. S., Brack, Ch., Sturm, R., Oberheuser, F. and Knuppen, R. (1990). Gonadotropin releasing hormone binding sites in human epithelial ovarian carcinomata. *Eur. J. Cancer Clin. Oncol.*, **25**, 215–221

63. Kullander, S. (1986). LH-RH agonist treatment in ovarian cancer. *Eur. J. Cancer Clin. Oncol.*, **22**, 724

64. Parmar, H., Nicoll, J., Stockdale, A., Cassoni, A., Phillips, R. H., Lightman, S. L. and Schally, A. V. (1985), Advanced ovarian carcinoma: response to the agonist D-Trp-6-LHRH. *Cancer Treatm. Rep.*, **69**, 1341–2

65. Parmar, H., Rustin, G., Lightman, S. L., Phillips, R. H., Hanham, I. W. and Schally, A. V. (1988). Response to D-Trp-6-luteinising hormone releasing hormone (Decapeptyl) microcapsules in advanced ovarian cancer. *Br. Med. J.*, **296**, 1229

66. Jäger, W., Wildt, L. and Lang, N. (1989). Observations on the course of advanced ovarian carcinomas after reduction of hypophyseal gonadotropins. *Geburtshilfe Frauenheilkd.*, **49**, 611–17

67. Kavanagh, J. J., Roberts, W., Townsend, P. and Hewitt, S. (1989). Leuprolide acetate in the treatment of refractory or persistent epithelial ovarian cancer. *J. Clin. Oncol.*, **7**, 115–18

68. Bruckner, H. W. and Motwani, B. T. (1989). Treatment of advanced refractory ovarian carcinoma with gonadotropin-releasing hormone analogue. *Am. J. Obstet. Gynecol.*, **161**, 1216–18

69. Emons, G., Pahwa, G. S., Ortamnn, O., Fassl, H., Löhrs, U., Schulz, K.-D. and Oberheuser, F. (1991). In Lunenfeld, B. (ed.) *GnRH Analogues and Cancer*, Vol 4. pp. 65–8. (Carnforth, UK: Parthenon Publishing)

70. Srkalovic, G., Wittliff, J. L. and Schally, A. V. (1990). Detection and partial characterization of receptors for (D-Trp-6)-luteinizing hormone releasing hormone and epidermal growth factor in human endometrial carcinoma. *Cancer Res.*, **50**, 1841–6

71. Gallagher, C. J., Oliver, R. T., Ohram, D. H., Fowler, C. G., Blake, P. R., Mantell, B. S., Slevin, M. L. and Hope-Stone, H. F. (1991). A new treatment for endometrial cancer with gonadotropin releasing-hormone analogue. *Br. J. Obstet. Gynaecol.*, **98**, 1037–41

BIBLIOGRAPHY

Abstracts of relevant papers presented at the 3rd International Symposium on GnRH Analogues in Cancer and Human Reproduction

114. Randomised trial comparing Zoladex with Nolvadex plus Zoladex in premenopausal advanced breast cancer. R. W. Blamey, UK

115. A phase II trial with D-Trp-6 (Decapeptyl) in premenopausal SAL RH +, hormonal untreated advanced breast cancer patients. T. Dorval, M. Jouve, A. Livartowski, T. Palangie, S. Scholl, P. Pouillart, France

117. Effect of Triptorelin (Decapeptyl) combined with heparin of estradiol levels in MCF-7 mammary cancer cells after incubation with estrone sulfate. J. R. Pasqualini, J. R. J. Blumberg-Tick, B. L. Nguyen, France

118. Inhibition of breast and endometrial cancer cell growth by the GnRH antagonist, SB-75, involves interference in IGFs autocrine/paracrine pathways. Y. Sharoni, D. Kleinman, E. Hershkovitz, M. Marback, E. Bosin, D. LeRoith, J. Levy, Israel

119. GnRH analogues and suppression of ovarian tumors – an experimental model. J. Blaakaer, M. Baksted, P. Albrectsen, J. Rygaard, J. Bock, Denmark

120. GnRH analogues as consolidation therapy in ovarian cancer. M. Holzinger, B. Tartacovsky, Israel

121. Gn-RH expression in human ovarian cancers: possible evidence for an autocrine regulation. T. Ohno, A. Imai, T. Tamaya, Japan

122. LHRH analogues in ovarian and endometrial cancer. G. Emons, O. Rotmann, A. V. Schally, K.-D. Schulz, USA

123. A randomized comparision of Decapeptyl and tamoxifen, as treatment of progressive ovarian cancer. W. Jäger, Germany

124. A phase II trial of D-Trp-6-LHRH (Decapeptyl) in pretreated patients with advanced epithelial ovarian cancer. N. Wigler, I. G. Ron, O. Merimsky, M. Inbar, S. Chaitchik, Israel

9

GnRH agonists and safety

K. Bühler

It is evident that gonadotropin releasing hormone (GnRH) agonists offer a fascinating and attractive medical alternative in the hormonal treatment of a great number of benign and malignant sex hormone-dependent diseases in various disciplines of medicine, such as endometriosis, uterine fibroids, polycystic ovarian disease, ovarian and breast cancer in gynecology, prostatic cancer in urology, and precocious puberty in pediatrics. More and more, the use of GnRH agonist has become common as an adjunctive therapy in assisted reproductive procedures and in gynecological surgery. Evaluation of a new and potent medication must include accurate understanding of the endocrinological and metabolic changes, and, in the sensitive field of reproductive medicine, exclusion of teratogenic effects. With all the potential of hormone treatment of sex steroid-dependent disorders, prolonged utilization may lead to metabolic disturbances. In this situation, not only the benefit considerations but also risk and safety considerations are very important.

All the effects of chronic GnRH agonist treatment can be explained by the suppression of synthesis and secretion of biologically active pituitary gonadotropins and the consequent decrease in gonadal activity. So, luteinizing hormone (LH) and follicle stimulating hormone (FSH) levels decrease to values compatible with the early follicular phase of the menstrual cycle, and estradiol serum concentrations fall sharply during the first 2 weeks of administration and remain within the range of the early follicular phase or at castration levels during the treatment period (Figure 1). If GnRH agonist is administered as a long-acting depot preparation, a more pronounced inhibition of steroidogenesis can be achieved compared to that reached with the daily application[1].

139

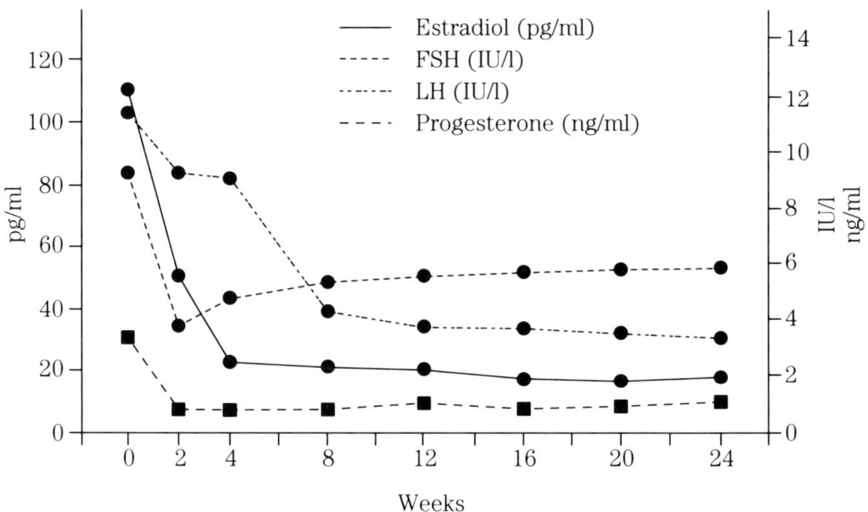

Figure 1 Hormonal changes during GnRH agonist treatment

The frequency and extent of side-effects, especially hot flushes, sweating and sleep disturbances, depend on estradiol levels: the lower the estradiol levels, the higher is the frequency of patients with side-effects (Figure 2). So, in a group of patients treated with GnRH agonists for uterine fibroids, 49% of the women complained of depression and 41% of headache before treatment was started, and in a group of patients treated for endometriosis, these rates were 64% and 47%, respectively.

The extent and frequency of other side-effects such as headache and depression depend more on personal conditions and less on hormonal alterations.

In summary, it could be demonstrated that extent and frequency of side-effects depend on the range of the estradiol deprivation, the duration of GnRH agonist treatment, the indication and the age of the patients.

With regard to the effects of GnRH treatment on blood chemistry, significant changes from pretreatment values could only be seen in hemoglobin blood levels in patients who were anemic prior to treatment (Figure 3) and in the alkaline phosphatase level.

It is well established that preoperative anemia is a major indication for intra- and postoperative blood transfusion in patients undergoing uterine surgery. Application of GnRH agonist prior to surgery in selected patients with uterine fibroids may decrease the need for blood transfusion,

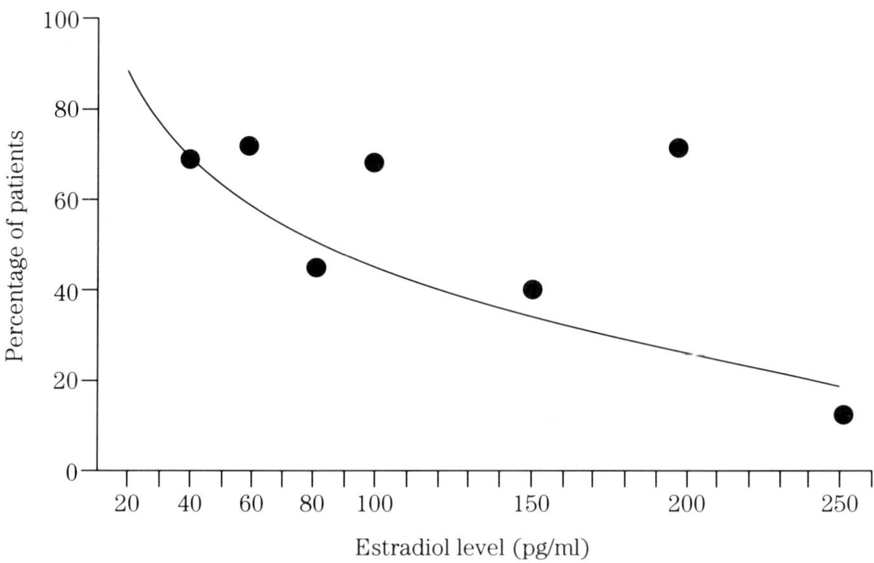

Figure 2 Frequencies of patients with hot flushes related to the estradiol level

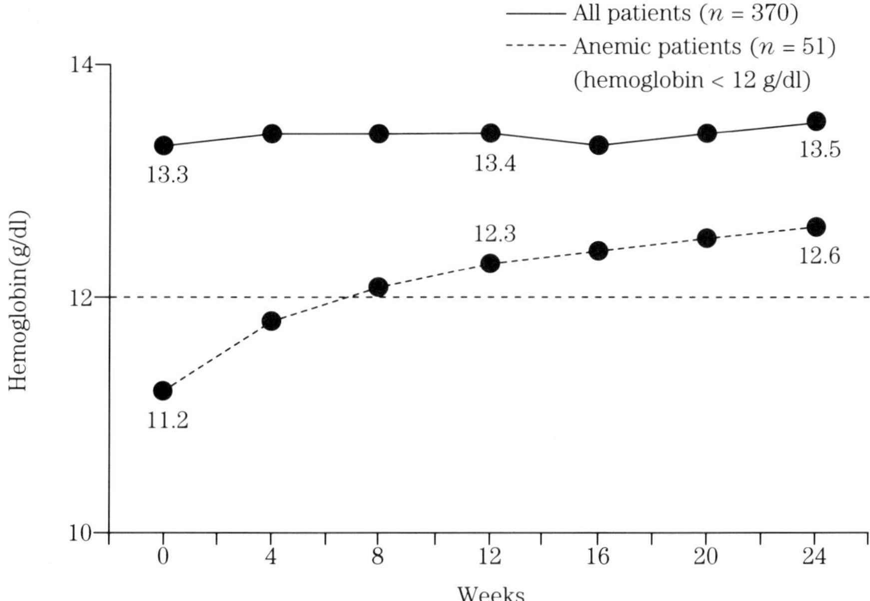

Figure 3 Hemoglobin blood level during GnRH agonist treatment, especially in anemic patients

by increasing the hemoglobin levels and because less blood is lost intraoperatively, since the uterine size is decreased and there are fewer surgical complications[2].

Although the increase of alkaline phosphatase is significant during GnRH agonist therapy, the level did not exceed the higher limit of the normal range[3]. This increase is due to the activation of bone metabolism. A 24-week treatment period with, for example, buserelin administration (900 µg/day intranasally) leads to a significant decrease in bone mineral density as compared with a control group [136]. There is a significant correlation between the differences in bone mineral density changes in the lumbar spine and the post-treatment estradiol level and the age of the patients. But as also found in other studies, bone loss was found to be reversible after agonist therapy was discontinued: 24 and 48 weeks after treatment, bone mineral density was not significantly different in the buserelin group and the control group. To prevent such a bone loss, especially in patients for whom long-term GnRH agonist application is required, e.g. premenstrual syndrome, selected cases of hirsutism, catamenial diseases like migraine and epilepsy, add-back treatments are becoming accepted [138]. When bone mineral density was compared after 1 year in patients receiving 0.625 mg or 1.25 mg of conjugated equine estrogen daily as adjunct to GnRH agonist, a significant and surprising 4% bone loss in the lumbar spine was seen with the lower dosage (higher dosage: +2%). Based on this observation, 1.25 mg of conjugated equine estrogen are recommended for estrogen add-back concomitant with GnRH agonist ovarian suppression [138]. Another approach to hormonal add-back therapy during GnRH agonist application is the use of tibolone (ORG OD14, 2.5 mg daily orally). Tibolone, a synthetic steroid with combined estrogenic, progestogenic and androgenic properties, has been shown to prevent post-menopausal bone loss[4] without stimulating the endometrium[5]. It could be shown that this steroid reduces significantly the bone mineral loss caused by GnRH agonist in the lumbar spine [139].

A further great advantage of such an add-back hormonal adjunct to GnRH agonist is demonstrated by the reduction of the vasomotor side-effects caused by the agonists. Patients receiving tibolone as add-back therapy showed a significantly lower frequency in hot flushes than patients treated with the GnRH agonist alone [140]. No differences could be seen after 6-month comparative treatment in the reduction of the American Fertility Society (AFS) scores; however, only a small number of patients with endometriosis ($n = 27$) was examined.

No changes could be observed in the levels of the liver enzymes SGOT, SGPT and γGT during a 6-month treatment with a GnRH agonist depot formulation.

Lipid metabolism is sensitive to changes in gonadal steroid levels and may be a good indicator of overall metabolic effects. Of primary interest is the fact that high plasma cholesterol levels seem to be the classical lipid risk factor for coronary heart disease. Leuprorelin treatment did not affect significantly either triglyceride or total cholesterol concentrations. Of greater interest concerning atherogenicity are the changes in high- (HDL) and low-density (LDL) lipoprotcins. In leuprorelin-treated patients, no significant change was observed in HDL and LDL concentrations. Both showed only a small increase during the treatment period, especially during the 1st month. Consequently, the LDL/HDL ratio did not change. This index is considered to be a good indicator of future risk of developing heart disease.

But what about the acute risk of thromboembolic complications? From the study of the effects of oral contraceptives, it is known that they affect the hemostasis system which, in some cases, may lead to fatal complications. The hemostasis system can be regarded as a dynamic balance of pro- and anti-coagulatory and pro- and antifibrinolytic activities. Under steady-state conditions, fibrin turnover, measured in D-dimer fibrin degradation products, is an excellent indicator of the activity of the actual hemostatic process.

In summary, three essential changes could be observed: procoagulant activity is significantly reduced; fibrinolytic reactivity shows a clear improvement and the fibrin turnover rate is significantly decreased, indicating a marked reduction in the rate of fibrin generation and degradation (Figure 4). The data suggest that GnRH agonist therapy may be beneficial in reducing the risk of thromboembolic disease. This will be important in patients undergoing surgery or prolonged bed-rest or with tumor-associated hypercoagulability[6].

In general, only a brief application of GnRH agonists is necessary for its adjuvant role in ovulation induction. In such a short course of therapy, hypoestrogenemia is not a concern. But, regarding other potentially negative effects on reproductive tissues and organs, above all, teratogenicity must be excluded. Various animal experimental studies have been undertaken to elucidate a possible deleterious influence on implantation and embryonal/fetal development. Indeed, in the rat, a pre- and postimplantational antifertility effect of agonists (pre- and postimplantory abortions, and very low fetal weight) was observed [137]. Vaginal application of the agonist, giving lower but much longer-sustained serum concentration levels, seems to be

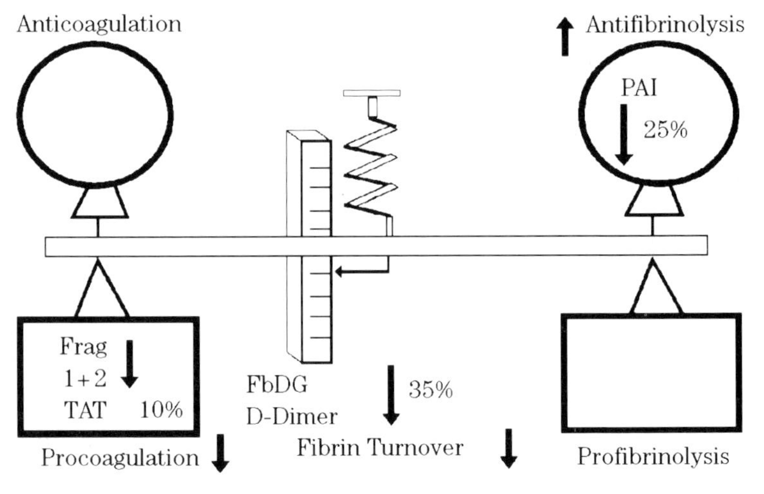

Figure 4   Model of the dynamic balance in hemostasis and the most important changes under GnRH agonist treatment[6]

more effective[7]. But one must take into consideration that the trophoblast function and its endocrinological regulation are completely different compared with the human system[8]. In the human, GnRH agonists given to women 5–8 weeks pregnant for 4–10 days did not lower human chorionic gonadotropin (hCG) or progesterone levels[9]. The fact that higher pregnancy and take-home-baby rates have been found in combined stimulation cycles (GnRH agonist + gonadotropins), especially in patients stimulated for assisted reproduction techniques, and the fact that the fetal outcome displays no difference with regard to the stimulation procedure used [79], suggest that persistence of minimal amounts of GnRH agonist, during the luteal phase, during the time of implantation and even during an early stage of pregnancy has no deleterious effect on oocyte quality, embryo viability and fetal well-being. Another cause for concern is the casual exposure to a GnRH agonist when pregnancy is not recognized at the first or repetitive application in a stimulation regimen, for endometriosis or fibroma. Twenty-four pregnancies were observed in which one to five injections of triptorelin depot formulation (3.75 mg) were administered up to the 21st week of amenorrhea [137]. The examination of the children suggests that triptorelin exerts no toxic or teratogenic effects in pregnant women. However, too few clinical cases were reported to enable a definite conclusion to be drawn and long-term follow-up should be undertaken in order to assess the impact of GnRH agonists on these children as they enter puberty.

GnRH agonists have a widespread applicability in a great variety of disorders and wide-scale clinical use has proven their efficacy. However, not only potency aspects are relevant; the safety of such powerful agents has to be proven too. As presented during the 3rd International Symposium on GnRH Analogues and currently reported in the literature, no apparent negative impacts of GnRH agonists could be established. However, a few questions should be answered in the future:

(1) No negative influence on oocyte quality, pregnancy rate and fetal outcome could be demonstrated. To discard the possibility of late side-effects of GnRH agonists applied during the postimplantation period or in early pregnancy, the offspring will have to be examined as they enter puberty.

(2) Considering that the reproductive phase of a woman's life is normally interrupted once or several times by shorter or longer states of hypoestrogenism due to lactation, the question arises if the importance of temporary bone loss caused by the 3–6-month application of GnRH agonists has a significant impact.

(3) Before add-back therapies are routinely introduced as an adjunct to GnRH agonist treatment, it must be proven in large prospective randomized trials that they do not reduce the efficacy of GnRH agonists.

All we can say today is that, measured with the highest available degrees of accuracy and sensitivity, and considering all their tremendous potential, GnRH agonists are safe and no really deleterious metabolic disturbances have been described as yet. As a result, these agents can continue to provide a revolutionary approach to and a manifold impact on the treatment of an increasing array of diseases.

REFERENCES

1. Bühler, K., Winkler, U., Scheit, S., Rempel, E. and Schindler, A. E. (1992). Different formulations of GnRH agonists in the treatment of endometriosis. In Lunenfeld, B. (ed.) *Advances in the Study of GnRH Analogues*, pp. 189–94. (Carnforth, UK: Parthenon Publishing)

2. Friedman, A. J. and Barbieri, R. L. (1988). Leuprolide acetate: applications in gynecology. *Curr. Probl. Obstet. Gynecol. Fertil.*, **11**, 205–36

3. Bühler, K., Winkler, U. and Schindler, A. E. (1992). Influence on hormone levels, lipid metabolism and reversibility of endocrinological changes after leuprorelin acetate depot therapy. *Clin. Therapeut.*, **14** (Suppl. a), 104–13

4. Lindsay, R., Hart, D. M. and Kraszewski, A. (1990). Prospective double-blind trial of synthetic steroid (Org OD14) for preventing postmenopausal osteoporosis. *Br. Med. J.*, **280**, 1207–9

5. Genazzani, A. R., Benedek-Jaszmann, L. J., Hart, D. M., Andolsek, L., Kicovic, P. M. and Tax, L. (1991). Org OD14 and the endometrium. *Maturitas*, **13**, 243–51

6. Winkler, U., Bühler, K., Koslowski, S., Oberhoff, C. and Schindler, A. E. (1992). Plasmatic haemostasis in gonadotrophin-releasing hormone analogue therapy: effects of leuprorelin acetate depot on coagulatory and fibrinolytic activities. *Clin. Therapeut.*, **14** (Suppl. a), 114–20

7. Yamazaki, I. (1982). Pregnancy terminating effect of a highly active LH-RH agonist by vaginal application in rats. *Endocrinol. Jpn.*, **29**, 197–207

8. Kato, K., Sairam, M. R. and Manjunath, P. (1983). Inhibition of implantation and termination of pregnancy in the rat by human chorionic gonadotropin antagonist. *Endocrinology*, **113**, 195–201

9. Sandow, J. (1983). Clinical applications of LHRH and its analogues. *Clin. Endocrinol.*, **18**, 571–92

BIBLIOGRAPHY

Abstracts of relevant papers presented at the 3rd International Symposium on GnRH Analogues in Cancer and Human Reproduction

79. Pregnancy outcome after GnRH-analogue/hMG therapy. W. Braendle, A. Kleinkauf-Houcken, S. Köhler, Ch. Lindner, Germany

135. Special aspects of side effects and blood chemistry during GnRHa treatment. K. Bühler, Germany

136. Bone mineral density (BMD) during and after ovarian suppression with a GnRH agonist. T. Uemera, T. Hirao, J. Mohri, H. Osada, N. Suzuki, N. Katagiri, H. Minaguchi, Japan

137. Follow-up of pregnancies after casual exposure to a GnRH analogue (triptorelin). C. Roux, E. Elefant, B. Biour, B. Schatz, France

138. 1.25 mg. of conjugated equine estrogen is preferable to 0.625 mg. for prevention of bone loss in GnRHa with hormonal add-back therapy. J. A. Nisker, A. Sugimoto, A. B. Hodsman, Canada

139. The effect of Org OD14 on GnRH agonist induced bone loss. P. C. Lindsay, R. W. Shaw, P. Kicovic, H. J. T. Coelingh Bennink, Great Britain/The Netherlands

140. ORG OD14 reduces the vasomotor side effects of GnRH agonists. P. C. Lindsay, K. G. Waller, R. W. Shaw, P. Kicovic, H. J. T. Coelingh Bennink, Great Britain/The Netherlands

10

Epilogue

B. Lunenfeld and V. Insler

The potency of gonadotropin releasing hormone (GnRH) and its analogues as stimulators, when administered in a precise pulsatile fashion, or inhibitors of pituitary gonadotropin secretion, when administered chronically, permits its use as an ovulation inducer on the one hand, and as a method of 'reversible medical gonadectomy' when applied to treatment of diseases dependent on gonadal steroids, on the other hand. Laboratory efforts in the synthesis of GnRH agonists have produced a large cluster of agents sufficient for practically all clinical purposes. The delivery systems, however, could still be improved to enable more convenient chronic application (oral, vaginal and, possibly, transdermal).

During the Third International Symposium on GnRH Analogues in Cancer and Human Reproduction held in Geneva, Switzerland in February 1993, the main chemical features of different GnRH agonists were presented. The reasons for the development of GnRH antagonists were discussed. The available new GnRH antagonists, their chemical properties and pharmacodynamic characteristics were described, and future developments were evaluated regarding optimal formulations and chemical structures tailor-made to specific GnRH receptors.

The state of the art of some specific clinical applications of GnRH agonists was presented. The rationale advantages and pitfalls of the use of agonists for the treatment of endometriosis, uterine fibroids and female infertility were discussed in detail.

The problem regarding safety of prolonged pituitary and ovarian suppression was perused from different angles, and various 'add-back' protocols were debated.

The advantages and disadvantages of agonists versus antagonists in future therapeutic regimens were explored. The avenues of future research concerning GnRH analogues (agonists and antagonists) were specified and some particular features were discussed in depth. Presentations and discussions at the Symposium permitted the formulation of future perspectives for research and applications of GnRH analogues.

The initial surge in luteinizing hormone/follicle stimulating hormone (LH/FSH) following GnRH agonist administration is an undesired side-effect, since clinically it is capable of causing a temporary flare-up of the disease. Additionally, agonists suppress sex steroids right down to the castrate level, and, as a result, chronic use (over 3–6 months) of agonists can cause bone loss. If partial suppression of sex steroids (for example in endometriosis) were attainable, this side-effect could be reduced. For these reasons, in the last 20 years scientists have searched for a potent and safe GnRH antagonist which would suppress LH/FSH secretion from the onset of treatment. Most importantly, the extent of suppression would be dose-dependent.

The necessary criteria for antagonist efficiency can now be defined more clearly. They are:

(1) High gonadotropin suppressive potency;

(2) Decreased complexity and increased ease of synthesis;

(3) Easy formulation in an aqueous vehicle (solubility) with none or low gelling effects. Gelling will give rise to a subcutaneous depot effect which may result in irritation at the site of injection and may cause random and mostly unpredictable release of the antagonist into the circulation;

(4) Low histamine release;

(5) Dose-dependent effect and controllable duration of action.

The recent cloning of the mouse[1] and human[2] GnRH receptors and elucidation of their sequences have elicited a great deal of scientific interest and activity, both in structural biology and in drug design. Using the published sequences, several laboratories have modeled the GnRH receptor and are trying to refine it experimentally. The model of the receptor structure will be utilized to design more efficient analogues as well as peptidomimetic or non-peptidic orally active antagonists.

Additional basic research concerning the biology of GnRH antagonists must be carried out. The binding and function of GnRH analogues in other organs as well as the pituitary have to be explored. Confirmation of recently produced experimental data could open new avenues for control of some malignant tumors, by application of specific GnRH antagonists[3]. An effort should also be made to discriminate between the actions of agonists and antagonists with respect to their effect on FSH and free α-subunit secretion, tumor cell proliferation and immune response.

A future therapy consisting of a combination of GnRH agonist and antagonist could be imagined in which the agonist would be used initially, to reduce pituitary gonadotrope receptors, and would be followed by administration of a smaller amount of antagonist, in order to obtain a subtle, exactly dose-dependent effect. In situations where chronic therapy is necessary and the initial flare-up harmful, a different type of combination therapy could also be imagined, in other words, initial suppression of gonadotropin activity by antagonist followed by continuous GnRH agonist application.

The value of GnRH agonists in the treatment of female infertility by using the induction of superovulation (controlled ovarian hyperstimulation) modality has proven to be impressive. By abolishing untimely LH surges, the combined pituitary suppression/ovarian stimulation therapy has significantly improved the pregnancy rates. This, however, was associated with longer duration of therapy and a higher dose requirement of gonadotropins.

Recent studies[4] have shown that a short-term application of GnRH antagonist, during a defined period of follicular development, prevented the appearance of a premature LH surge, thus allowing complete follicular maturation prior to the triggering of ovulation with hCG. This type of combined therapy could obviously offset the objectionable features of GnRH agonist/gonadotropin treatment. Furthermore, a sequential treatment, consisting of pituitary–ovarian suppression by a GnRH antagonist followed by induction of follicular growth by pulsatile GnRH, can also be imagined.

It is fascinating to recall that one of the major rationales for the development of GnRH analogues was male and female contraception. After 20 years of effort and trial, today there are still no sufficient data to determine whether application of GnRH agonists or antagonists for this indication is efficient, safe, acceptable and economical.

Taking into account the difficulties encountered in devising effective, safe and simple-to-produce GnRH antagonists, the question arises whether such agents are really needed for clinical use and, if yes, what are the exact indications for their application? It seems that antagonists would be required:

(1) In all clinical situations where the flare-up has a pronounced negative effect;

(2) Where the suppressing effect is required to appear immediately after administration;

(3) In situations when the suppressive effect has to be exactly controlled;

(4) In situations where immediate reversal of the suppressive effect (by pulsatile GnRH application) is necessary.

None of the GnRH agonists or antagonists which have been clinically tested were capable of total suppression of LH or FSH. It is, however, uncertain whether such preparations can be devised and questionable whether they would be of any practical benefit.

The Third International Symposium on GnRH Analogues in Cancer and Human Reproduction held in Geneva, Switzerland in February 1993 has demonstrated that significant advances have been made in the understanding of the mechanisms and effects of GnRH analogues in the diagnosis and treatment of many pathological conditions. For the participants, this book should provide a summary of the presentations, discussions and ideas. For all readers, it should serve as a short and concise compendium of the state of art in 1993.

We do hope that this volume will stimulate scientists and clinicians throughout the world to continue their efforts in exploiting the potential of GnRH agonists and antagonists to be diagnostic and therapeutic tools. Their success in accomplishing this task will become evident a the Fourth International Symposium, February 8–11, 1996. We hope to meet you then, as usual, at the Intercontinental Hotel in Geneva, Switzerland.

REFERENCES

1. Tsutsumi, M., Zhou, W., Miller, R. P., Mellon, P. L., Roberts, J. L., Flanagan, C. A., Dong, K., Gillo, B. and Sealfon, S. (1992). Cloning and functional expression of a mouse gonadotropin-releasing hormone receptor. *Mol. Endocrinol.*, **6**, 1163–9
2. Kaker, S. S., Musgrove, L. C., Devor, D. C., Sellers, J. C. and Neill, J. D. (1992). Cloning, sequencing, and expression of human gonadotropin releasing hormone (GnRH) receptor. *Biochem. Biophys. Res. Commun.*, **171**, 289–95
3. Sharoni, Y., Kleinman, D., Hershkovitz, E., Marbach, M., Bozin, E., LeRoith, D. and Levy, J. (1993). Inhibition of yeast and endometrial cancer cell growth by the

GnRH antagonist SB-75 involves interference in IGFs autocrine–paracrine pathways. *Gynecol. Endocrinol.*, **7** (Suppl. 1), in press

4. Bouchard, Ph., Dubourdieu, Frydman, R. and Charbonnel, B. (1993). GnRH antagonist administration during the periovulatory period prevents LH surges in normal women: a possible role for GnRH antagonists in controlled ovarian stimulation. *Gynecol. Endocrinol.*, **1** (Suppl. 1), in press

Index

add-back therapy using GnRH
    agonist 51
  staging classification 49
β-endorphin 38–9
EP24 332 14
epidermal growth factor 59
epilepsy 142
erythema 21
estradiol 38–9, 58, 59
estriol 73
estrogens 124
  cardiovascular complications 104
estrone 58
ethinylestradiol 73

female infertility treatment 37–46
  comparison of protocols for
    pituitary suppression 42–3
  congenital malformations
    following 42
fibrin turnover 143, 144
fibroids *see* uterine leiomyomata
Flutamide 104, 107, 108–18
follicle stimulating hormone 27, 31,
  139, 148
  inhibition 18
folligen 127–8
forskolin 32

Ganirdix 14, 20
gel formation 15, 16
gestrinone 50, 62
glucose-6-phosphate dehydrogenase
  56
GnRH analogues 13–20
  biological properties 15
  anti-fertility effect 143–4
  anti-tumor activity 19
  biological actions 18
  castration effect 103–4

cytotoxic analogues 128–9
depot preparations 139, 143
duration of action 16
efficiency criteria 148
half-lifes 16
physical properties 15
short-time application 149
side-effects 140–5
gonadal steroids 29
gonadotropin release/synthesis 27–33
  biosynthesis 31–2
gonadotropin releasing hormone 27–8
gonadotropin theory 129
goserelin 37, 41, 63, 113, 125–6
  for leiomyomata 71
  plus tamoxifen 126–7
gossypol 62
G protein 28, 29
growth hormone 38–9
GTP-binding protein 33

hemoglobin 141, 142
hirsutism 142
histamine release activity 17, 22
human chorionic gonadotropin 43
human GnRH receptor cloning 148
human placental lactogen 59
hydrocortisone 124
hydrophilic/hydrophobic peptides
  15–16
4-hydroxyandrostenedione 126–7
hypoestrogenemia 143

incessant ovulation hypothesis 129
inhibins 27
inositol phosphate 128
inositol-1,4,5-triphosphate 33
insulin-like growth factor-1 38–9, 128
ionomycin 32
in vitro fertilization 18